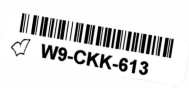

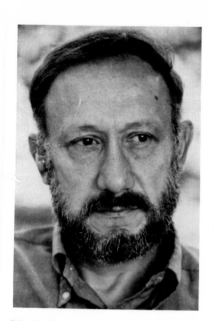

HARD OF HEARING CHILDREN IN REGULAR SCHOOLS

Mark Ross, Ph.D., Professor of Audiology at the University of Connecticut, has written over fifty articles and chapters and has participated widely in professional meetings and workshops.

Diane Brackett, Ph.D., and Antonia Maxon, Ph.D. are co-directors of the UCONN Mainstream project, concerning hard of hearing children in regular schools.

REMEDIATION OF COMMUNICATION DISORDERS SERIES

Frederick N. Martin, Series Editor

STUTTERING

Edward G. Conture

HEARING IMPAIRMENTS IN YOUNG CHILDREN

Arthur Boothroyd

HARD OF HEARING CHILDREN IN REGULAR SCHOOLS

Mark Ross with Diane Brackett and Antonia Maxon

HEARING-HANDICAPPED ADULTS

Thomas G. Giolas

ACQUIRED NEUROGENIC DISORDERS

Thomas P. Marquardt

LANGUAGE DISORDERS IN PRESCHOOL CHILDREN

Patricia R. Cole

LANGUAGE DISORDERS IN SCHOOL AGE CHILDREN

Mary Lovey Wood

Forthcoming

ARTICULATION DISORDERS

Ronald K. Sommers

CEREBRAL PALSY

James C. Hardy

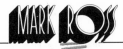

with Diane Brackett and Antonia Maxon

University of Connecticut

HARD OF HEARING CHILDREN IN REGULAR SCHOOLS

Prentice-Hall, Inc., Englewood Cliffs, New Jersey 07632

Library of Congress Cataloging in Publication Data

Ross, Mark.
    Hard of hearing children in regular schools.
    (Remediation of communication disorders)
    Bibliography: p.
    Includes index.
    1. Hearing impaired children—Education.
2. Mainstreaming in education. 3. Remedial
teaching. I. Brackett, Diane. II. Maxon,
Antonia. III. Title. IV. Series.
HV2437.R67   371.91'2   81-13898
ISBN 0-13-383802-1   AACR2

©1982 by Prentice-Hall, Inc., Englewood Cliffs, N.J. 07632

Printed in the United States of America

10 9 8 7 6 5 4 3 2 1

Editorial/production supervision by Virginia Cavanagh Neri
Interior design by Maureen Olsen
Cover design by Maureen Olsen
Manufacturing buyer: Edmund W. Leone
Author's photo by William Rubens

ISBN 0-13-383802-1

Prentice-Hall International, Inc., *London*
Prentice-Hall of Australia Pty. Limited, *Sydney*
Prentice-Hall of Canada, Ltd., *Toronto*
Prentice-Hall of India Private Limited, *New Delhi*
Prentice-Hall of Japan, Inc., *Tokyo*
Prentice-Hall of Southeast Asia Pte. Ltd., *Singapore*
Whitehall Books Limited, *Wellington, New Zealand*

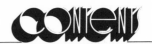

Contents

Foreword ix

Preface xi

One

Hard of hearing children in regular schools 1

Two

Performance of the hard hearing child 15

Evaluation of the hard of hearing child 52

Remediation 126

Appendix 233

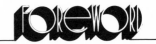

With the information explosion of recent years there has been a proliferation of knowledge in the areas of scientific and social inquiry. The speciality of communicative disorders has been no exception. While two decades ago a single textbook or "handbook" might have sufficed to provide the aspiring or practicing clinician with enlightenment on an array of communication handicaps, this is no longer possible—hence the decision to prepare a series of single-author texts.

As the title implies, the emphasis of this series, *Remediation of Communication Disorders,* is on therapy and treatment. The authors of each book were asked to provide information relative to anatomical and physiological aspects of each disorder, as well as pathology, etiology, and diagnosis to the extent that an understanding of these factors bears on management procedures. In such relatively short books this was quite a challenge: to offer guidance without writing a "cookbook"; to be selective without being parochial; to offer theory without losing sight of practice. To this challenge the series' authors have risen magnificently.

My friendship with Mark Ross goes back over twenty-five years, when we were undergraduate and later graduate students together. His interest in hearing disorders goes back even further than that as a result of a hearing loss first manifest in young adulthood. As a student, he was *always* a top scholar, with predictions from professors and peers alike that he would make a bold and indelible mark on the profession of audiology. Even before completion of his graduate work, he had begun to earn a reputation as an expert in aural rehabilitation. After establishing himself as a professor at the University of Connecticut, Dr. Ross was impelled by his sense of dedication to leave the security of academia—to which he has since returned—to assume the directorship of a school for the deaf. To this position he took the insights and innovations expressed in this book, which were later intensified and enlarged by his experiences at the school and reflected in these pages. This book also reflects the contributions of his two colleagues, Drs. Diane Brackett and Antonia Maxon, codirectors of the UConn Mainstream Project, who have drawn liberally upon their widespread experiences in the project. Together, they have created a complete and important volume in the management of hearing-impaired children.

FREDERICK N. MARTIN
Series Editor

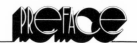

The first words of this book were written several years after Public Law 94-142 had been in full force. This law, the Education for All Handicapped Children Act, brought in its wake a great deal of confusion, bureaucratic wrinkles to iron out, and what appears to have been a complete reorganization of special education in the United States. We have, in the pages to follow, expressed some reservations from time to time on how the law was actually being implemented at the grass roots level though we have fully supported its basic intentions. These present words are being written at a time (August 1981) while the future of the law is being debated at the highest educational levels in our country. Some of the information we have received suggests that either outright repeal of the law is being sought or, at the least, a severe gutting of its mandatory provisions.

In spite of our reservations about Public Law 94-142, we do not feel it is possible to turn the clock backwards in respect to the total educational management of hard of hearing children. Special educators at all levels are learning how to implement the spirit of the law in a more efficient manner. Children who were never serviced or who were underserviced for special needs are now on therapy or tutorial rolls; parents have learned that the Federal Government stands behind them in their efforts to secure adequate educational provisions for their children, and a massive in-service training program has been in effect for regular and special educators. From our perspective, some progress has been made—though few would disagree that much remains to be done. We think it would be a serious mistake to weaken or eliminate the law now.

If this were done, the education of all children with special needs would again be thrown into confusion. To withdraw services from children that were once available would not only be cruel, but uneconomical as well. Our primary goal in special education, at least with hearing-impaired children whom we know best, is to assist these youngsters to develop into economically self-sufficient adults. We have in the following pages amply documented the educational gaps manifested by these children which occur as a direct result of their hearing impairment. We have also presented material on how this gap can be reduced or eliminated with an effective (broadly defined) educational program. To try to save money in the short run by reducing such services to these children—and in spite of the verbiage to the contrary this would be the inevitable result of repealing or eliminating the mandatory provisions of PL 94-142—is to continue to raise a generation of underemployed and underachieving hard of hearing children, with a greater long term burden on the society as a whole.

Let us, however, continue to be optimistic. Whatever happens to PL 94-142, hard of hearing children are going to be with us, and they are going to have to be educated. Of all the children with special needs, hard of hearing children, in our judgment, have the best prognosis for improvement. We know the cause of their problem, we know that its genesis is their ears and not their brain, and we know much about how to circumvent their basic problem by employing their residual hearing to the fullest extent. In working with hard of hearing children, our greatest ally is their normal biological capacity for developing speech and language, given a sufficient quantity of exposure to the language at appropriate times. We have, therefore, stressed an auditory management approach to these children as the best method of capitalizing on their innate capacities, but not to the exclusion of more traditional speech and language and classroom management procedures.

We have also stressed a comprehensive performance evaluation, which includes not just an audiological work-up, but the most complete inventory we can manage of their communication skills. An organized program of therapy is not possible if we are unable to define the children's strengths and weaknesses. One component of this performance evaluation is a detailed classroom observation. For most children, this is the pay off. How they learn and adapt in and to a regular classroom is a crucial standard which must be applied to them. A child's physical placement in a regular classroom is not in itself a criteria of a successful educational effort; "mainstreaming" per se simply informs us where the children are being educated, not how well this is being done.

To do the best job possible with hard of hearing children, with or without PL 94-142, the professionals who work with them must not only master a body of information—the purpose of this book—but must also take on the role of a somewhat zealous missionary. Hard of hearing children are a misunderstood minority in our schools. To those who do not understand the varying effects of different degrees and types of hearing losses, their behavior is frequently misunderstood and often condemned. The speech-language pathologist, audiologist, or teacher of the hearing impaired who is serving as a primary support person for these children has to act as their major professional advocate in the schools. They have to assist the regular teachers and the other personnel to interpret the children's behavior correctly and convey to them concrete management suggestions, all of this in the spirit of a colleague and not a critic. Often they have to recommend expensive amplification systems for the children, incurring the wrath of budget minded administrators when they do. They should see themselves as having no choice but to forcefully advocate what must be done if the children are to realize their potential. It is not an easy job, but for the professionals who measure their worth in terms of their effectiveness, their efforts are crowned with success often enough to make the job eminently rewarding.

Much of this book was written while the senior author was on sabbatical leave at the Program for the Hearing Impaired in Tel Aviv University in Israel. Dr. Jerome Reichstein, head of the program and a good friend and colleague, was most helpful in his comments and assistance throughout. This is a new program, the first of its kind in the country, and in developing a curriculum and practicum experiences to train students to work with both the deaf and hard of hearing populations, the issues and problems faced in Israel helped in the development of the approach taken in this book.

We would also like to acknowledge the contribution of the many children and professionals we have worked with during our federally funded UConn Mainstream Project. In the past five years, we have conducted an in-service training program for professionals who work with hearing-impaired children in the regular schools. The insights we have gained during this period are contained in the following pages.

Most of all, we want to convey our appreciation to the children we have seen. They are our charge and our blessing, and our fervent hope is that we have done them justice in the writing of this book.

MARK ROSS
DIANE BRACKETT
ANTONIA MAXON

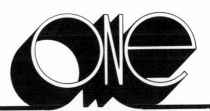

Hard of hearing children in regular schools

○ INTRODUCTION

This book is devoted specifically to the habilitation of the hard of hearing child in a regular school setting. By clearly defining the theme and thrust of the book, we hope to preclude many of the conceptual confusions that have weakened much of the previous literature on this topic. The book is not about "deaf" but "hard of hearing" children. It is a distinction that has been made on a number of previous occasions (Ross and Calvert 1967; Wilson, Ross, and Calvert 1974; Ross and Giolas 1978) and, though it may be repetitious to keep on making it, it is nevertheless of continuing relevance to the education of children with hearing losses. Professionals charged with providing direct or supportive services to these children must understand this distinction in order to manage their habilitative needs in an intelligent and effective manner. Simply said, the first step in dealing with any disorder is to understand it.

The content level of the book assumes that the reader has had introductory courses in speech, language, and audiology. The book is not designed for persons with no, or extremely limited, pertinent academic background, but rather for speech-language pathologists, educational audiologists, and teachers of the hearing-impaired who work, or are in training to work, with hard of hearing children in the regular schools.

the hard of hearing child

The hard of hearing child is developing, or has developed, his basic communication skills through the auditory channel. His residual hearing is sufficient, with or without amplification, to serve as the basis for his evolving speech and language skills. Although these skills are more often deficient than not, he is, nonetheless, basically an auditory rather than a visual communicator. Thus he has much more in common with a normally hearing child than he does with a deaf child. And there are more hard of hearing than deaf children. The number of hard of hearing children in our school population with average losses in the better ear between 26 and 70 dB has been estimated at 1.6% (Public Health Service Publication, No. 1227, 43–44, 1964), or 16 per 1000 school children.

This incidence figure is frequently quoted; however, the evidence indicates that it minimizes the actual frequency of educationally significant disorders (defined to include speech, language, academic, and psycho-social disturbances attributable to the hearing loss). We know that the percentage of school children manifesting a hearing disorder increases with decreasing degree of loss. We also know that hearing losses in the 15 to 26 dB range are related to academic achievement lags in excess of one year (Quigley 1978, p. 43). Thus it follows that the actual percentage of children with educationally significant hearing losses is in excess of 16 per 1000, probably much closer to 30 per 1000.

We would consider any child with an average hearing loss of 16 dB or more in his better ear to be potentially "at risk" in regard to manifesting deficiencies associated with his hearing loss. In our judgment, this is the cut-off that should be used in separating the hard of hearing child from the normally hearing child. (The reader should understand that this classification is for categorical and labeling purposes only; individual children should always be dealt with on their own terms primarily, and only secondarily as a member of some category.)

the deaf child

In contrast to the hard of hearing child, the deaf child's development of speech and language, and his primary avenue of communication, are visually based. There is a world of difference between a group which communicates mainly through a visual mode (lipreading or manual communication) and one which communicates primarily through an auditory mode (albeit imperfectly). We have too often been beguiled by the apparent similarities between these two groups—after all, they both have hearing losses —and have ignored the profound differences implicit in the different channels they use to process primary sensory input. Lumping these two groups of children together has been a disservice to both, but mainly to the hard of hearing child. We find children who are, or were, potentially hard of hearing in just about every deaf education program in the country. Classified as "deaf," treated and educated as if they were "deaf," they do in fact function as deaf individuals (Ross and Calvert 1967). We do not mean to denigrate deaf individuals in any way by this statement. Our intention is to emphasize that the sense of hearing and its function in human beings is literally a human birthright, and professionals who ignore its presence in children are violating an important portion of the human potential.

It is as difficult to specify the physiological borderline between the "deaf" and "hard of hearing" as it is to divide the normally hearing from the hard of hearing listener. Functional descriptions—that is, how a person actually uses his hearing—would be the most valid method if we had the appropriate techniques, which we do not. A rough physiological separation between the potentially hard of hearing and the potentially deaf would be a hearing loss of 95 dB or more averaged across the speech frequencies (much of the evidence supporting this assertion is reviewed in Stark 1974). The demographic data regarding the incidence of congenital deafness is approximately one such individual per 1000 births. Thus there are 16 to 30 times fewer deaf children than hard of hearing ones.

We hasten to disabuse here the notion that deaf children, as they have been defined above, cannot use their residual hearing meaningfully. With very little residual hearing, deaf children can still perceive and produce the prosodic features of speech, identify the manner of articulation of a number of phonemes, and respond to the emotional intent of a speaker's message (Ross et al. 1973). Valuable as this information is for them, however, audition is still a secondary and supplemental channel to vision.

the in-between child

Obviously, not every hearing-impaired* child will be able to be neatly classified in one or the other of these categories. Some children with moderate losses apparently depend less upon their hearing than their vision, while others with severe losses appear to use their hearing as a primary channel on at least an equal basis with the visual channel (Seewald and Ross 1978). Our view is that there are understandable auditory reasons for these events, and that esoteric, abstract, and confusing diagnostic labels need not be invoked to explain these seemingly contradictory behaviors. These reasons will be fully developed below.

There are, nevertheless, numbers of children who, for whatever reasons, fall on the border line between the deaf and hard of hearing categories. They can utilize their hearing, derive much benefit from it, and may even employ it as a primary channel in certain restricted circumstances, when they have no other choice, such as talking on the telephone on a specific topic. At other times, they may prefer to depend primarily on the visual channel for communicative purposes. Performance and management generalizations about such children should be made very cautiously. We should keep in mind, however, that such children are relatively few in comparison to the entire population of hearing-impaired children. The overwhelming majority of hearing-impaired children, the ones with whom this book is primarily concerned, are, or could be, unquestionably hard of hearing who process information primarily via the auditory channel. We should not permit the ambiguous performance of a relatively few "borderline" children to blind us to this fact. We should not permit the clear conceptualization and therapeutic implications of the hard of hearing condition to be diverted by the occasional exceptions.

*The term "hearing-impaired" will be used in this book in a generic sense, to refer to all children with hearing losses, whether deaf or hard of hearing. Occasionally, such adjectives as "severe," "moderate," or "mild" will be used to qualify the term. Our goal is to be as precise in our description of the children as we can.

sensory deprivation

The necessity for the early detection of a hearing impairment now appears beyond dispute. Mechanisms have varied from mass hearing screening of the neonatal and infant populations to "high-risk" registers wherein only those children with certain histories or conditions are screened (Northern and Downs 1978; Martin 1978). A great deal of research has been generated to determine the most cost-effective methods of early detection of hearing loss, and in some states and localities laws and regulations have been promulgated requiring one or another hearing screening procedure be implemented. However, we would venture to guess that relatively few individuals supporting or engaged in such activities really understand why they are doing what they are doing, beyond such hazy notions as "the earlier we start the better." This is not enough. There are excellent and very supportable reasons why we must detect the presence of a hearing impairment early in the life of a child. Understanding these reasons will lend urgency to the efforts of those working for the early detection and management of hearing loss in children.

First, and perhaps foremost, is the necessity to preclude the occurrence of auditory sensory deprivation. We have known for many years about the deleterious effects of visual sensory deprivation in both animals and humans (reviewed in Katz 1978; and Kessler 1978). Although the analogy with auditory deprivation appears straightforward, it has been drawn only occasionally and with trepidation. Seeing is not hearing and what is true for one modality may not be true for the other. In recent years, however, there have been a number of studies on auditory deprivation, but only with animals. Though the detail effects will undoubtedly differ, there is no reason to believe that the major consequences of auditory deprivation with animals will not also be verified in human beings.

Rats temporarily deprived of sound during the first few months of life demonstrate a marked inferiority in responding to differences in sound patterns, attributed in large part by their inability to resolve time differences, though they show no such inferiority in simpler auditory dimensions (Tees 1967; Patchett 1977). A speech signal, we should recall, is a complex, patterned, acoustic event in which time differentiation plays a major role in its decoding. Other studies with rats have shown that early auditory deprivation increases the latency of auditory neural responses by a factor of 2 to 3 (Clopton and Winfield 1976), and that this sound deprivation produces morphologic changes in the brain stem auditory nuclei (Webster and Webster 1977). Chickens deprived of sound from the time of hatching (actually before, inasmuch as the ears of the embryonic chicks were occluded while they were still in the egg), demonstrate abnormal relationships between the

5

intensity of an input sound and the amplitude of the neural response. Abnormal binaural interaction effects have also been demonstrated at the mid-brain level after monaural deprivation (Silverman and Clopton 1977; Clopton and Silverman 1977).

All the research on this topic supports the general conclusion that depriving an animal of sound for some duration at an early period in its life will result in abnormalities in some auditory dimension. As stated earlier, there is no reason to believe that analogous effects do not occur with humans.

Fortunately (or perhaps unfortunately), we do have an accumulating body of evidence with humans on the effect of temporary auditory deprivation, a kind of "natural" experiment similar to the occurrence of congenital cataracts. We are referring to the occurrence in young children of middle ear problems that are usually, but not always, cleared up as the children get older. There have been a number of studies and clinical observations on this topic (reviewed in Katz 1978; and Kessler and Randolph 1979). In the Kessler study, two groups of third-grade children were compared, one with and one without a history of otitis media prior to age three. The results indicated that the experimental group was poorer than the control group in a number of auditory processing tasks, that their academic achievements were generally poorer than the control group, and that they were the recipients of significantly more remedial services than the control group.

Other studies on this same topic lend unambiguous support to this same conclusion (Holm and Kunze 1969; Hamilton and Owrid 1974; Dalzell and Owrid 1976; Needleman 1977; Zincus et al. 1978; Masters and Marsh 1978; Gottlieb et al. 1978; Zinkus and Gottlieb 1980)—namely, that children with early histories of otitis media demonstrate significant deficiencies in auditory sequential memory, phonemic synthesis, reading, phonology, and language skills. We should note that children with congenital sensorineural hearing losses, whose first experience with amplification is delayed until they are two or three years old are deprived of sound much more completely and consistently than children with fluctuating middle ear problems.

What this overbrief excursion on this topic should communicate to us is that if the auditory system does not experience some critical quantity of meaningful, patterned sound at some early period after birth, the system will demonstrate certain morphological and physiological abnormalities that will forever limit its performance below what it might have been. Roughly speaking, the evidence suggests that the earlier the deprivation occurs and the longer it lasts, the greater will be the deprivation effects. To end this section on a hopeful note, some restoration of auditory functions should always be possible, no matter how long the deprivation has lasted. Hearing aids have been recommended for congenitally, severely hearing-impaired adults and they have been delighted in being able to detect the presence of sounds and certain other gross acoustic dimensions. What is probable, however, in these instances, is that if amplification had been used when they were young, their auditory capability would have permitted them to distinguish spectral, as well as the wave envelope changes, in the auditory signal.

the "critical" period for speech and language development

Related to, but separate from, our concern with preventing auditory sensory deprivation is the concept of the critical, sensitive period for speech and language development (Lenneberg 1967). Our primary reason for attempting to preclude the occurrence of sensory deprivation is to permit the auditory channel to play its natural role in speech and language development. Given the existence of a functioning (albeit impaired) auditory channel, the growing child possesses an awesome capacity for organizing language inputs into a complex, rapidly evolving, oral language system. In the absence of an adequate auditory channel, the child would evolve a visually oriented system; the point is the child's early "predisposition" and capacity to develop a cognitively based and meaningful communication system. For the hard of hearing child, this capacity is most effectively associated with the use of residual hearing. Early detection and management will ensure both the preclusion of sensory deprivation and the appropriate timing for taking advantage of the child's maximum readiness period for speech and language development.

The point that we want to emphasize here is that the hard of hearing child possesses the same biological capacity for learning language as does the normally hearing child. In order for him to use this capacity, however, he requires exposure to an auditory sample of the language in relevant interpersonal situations. Because he has a hearing loss, because certain acoustic cues in speech will not be available to him, he needs more exposure to an auditory sample of the language than does a normally hearing person. There is nothing better that we can do for a hard of hearing child, in respect to his speech and language development, than to ensure that his biological capacity for learning language is maximally exploited by the effective use of amplified sound. We should not make the mistake of thinking that we are better teachers of language, with all our pedogogical efforts, than the child is a learner, with the assistance of his innate biological potential.

overlaid behavioral anomolies

The hard of hearing child presents a very confusing picture if one is not aware of the existence or effects of a hearing loss. On the one hand, he is not deaf; he does "hear" and respond appropriately to sounds and speech. On the other hand, his hearing loss prevents him from responding normally and consistently to these stimuli. Without an awareness of the presence and implications of a hearing loss, he is often considred somewhat "odd," negative, retarded, brain damaged, emotionally disturbed, and so on (Rosenberg 1965; Ross and Matkin 1967; Klefner 1973). His hearing loss may be detected later than deafness in deaf children, and he may be fitted with amplification and enrolled in an appropriate educational program much later than are deaf children (Elliot and Armbruster 1967). By the time the hearing loss is detected, or its effects understood by the significant persons in the child's life, he has already lived with the burden of being considered different—and been responded to in this fashion. Hard of hearing children may manifest a number of behavioral anomolies that appear coequal with the hearing impairment (Ross 1978). Professionals dealing with such a child should realize the strong possibility that these anomolies are really secondary problems—that is, responses of the child to being treated differently and to different expectations—which is not to deny their reality. Treatment of these overlaid problems must reflect an awareness of their possible genesis.

○ OVERVIEW OF INTERVENTION STRATEGIES

Although this book is devoted to the school-age hard of hearing child, we want to stress once again the imperatives of early detection and management. If the hearing loss is not detected in the very early years, if appropriate amplification techniques are not applied soon after detection, if the child is not enrolled in a suitable parent-infant or nursery program (see Boothroyd 1982), then the effectiveness of efforts with the older school-age child will undoubtedly be lessened. Nevertheless, whether the child is a recipient of early management procedures or not, he is still with us, he requires our help, and there is still much we can do for him.

Dealing with a hard of hearing child, our first need is to understand the nature and effect of his hearing impairment, which implies a comprehensive and continuing audiological evaluation. Pediatric and otological examinations are of course an absolute requirement. Given the existence of either a chronic middle ear problem or a permanent sensorineural hearing loss, however, the communicative, educational, and psycho-social effects of the hearing loss demand an explicit focus separate from the purely medical implications of the hearing impairment.

No nonmedical intervention strategy can be maximally effective unless the child receives a comprehensive performance evaluation. Such an evaluation includes an analysis of his (a) oral communication skills, both expressive and receptive; (b) language status, including the morphological, syntactical, semantic, and pragmatic components; (c) an intellectual evaluation, which must include an individually administered nonverbal component; (d) an academic achievement test battery; (e) classroom observations to judge its appropriateness for the child; (f) his psycho-social status in the school; (g) personal conferences with all the professional school personnel who come in contact with the child; and (h) finally, and of profound importance, conferences with the child's parents. The child's total educational program is planned on the basis of the unique constellation of performances and needs he displays in this comprehensive evaluation.

Given the fact that children are handicapped and are our concern because they manifest a hearing loss, the first steps that must be taken in managing their educational needs revolve around auditory factors. Careful auditory management can reduce the impact of the problem at its source—namely, the hearing impairment. This is not just another intervention factor among many others, to be taken care of before moving on to the next item. The child's language and speech skills reflect to a great extent his auditory status. It follows, therefore, that the more effectively he can utilize his residual hearing, the less deviant his communication abilities. In the classroom, his comprehension of the material will likewise reflect what he hears; the better he hears the teacher, the more he is likely to learn the material being presented. Thus, our first priority in managing a hard of hearing child in the regular schools is to ensure that he is using his hearing as effectively as possible.

We are not so naive as to believe that, with even the most perfectly arranged audiological management, we can eliminate the problems of most hard of hearing children. We can for *some* children, provided we begin early and do most things right. Nevertheless, for the majority of hard of hearing children, we are not going to eliminate all of their problems. We can, however, markedly reduce their severity and impact.

When we have done, and are continuing to do, all we can for a child with regard to audiological management, then our attention must be given to the residual educational effects of the hearing loss. We are defining "educational" in this context to include speech, language, and psycho-social factors. Of course, both audiological and educational management can, and often should, proceed concurrently; the point here is that audiological factors require the initial emphasis in management focus and will pay the greatest initial dividends in terms of a child's progress.

We visualize a preeminent role for the speech-language pathologist, and the educational audiologist, in regard to the hard of hearing child in the regular schools. In our judgment, those who possess the American Speech, Language-Hearing Association standards for certification, or its equivalent, possess the basic skills and background to serve as the "case coordinator" for the mainstreamed hard of hearing child. The training of these specialists in the basic and clinical aspects of communication disorders is directly transferable to the skills necessary to evaluate and manage the primary handicap these children display—their communication disorder—and its implications on their educational and psycho-social status.

To be sure, additional skills and information are necessary—indeed that is the purpose of this book—and these specialists are not going to do it alone. However, someone in the public schools has to serve as the resident "expert" regarding the educational programing of these children. In our estimation, this should be the qualified speech-language pathologist or the educational audiologist. (In many instances, this role can be filled by the teacher of the hearing impaired; generally speaking, however, the training of these individuals is more appropriate for working with the deaf rather than the hard of hearing child. Many, however, are eminently suited to fulfill this role.) Whichever professional assumes this role—and later we shall voice and justify our preference for the educational audiologist when both are available in the same school system—this is the one who must coordinate the diverse contributions of a number of specialists in the schools, organize and schedule educational planning meetings, and work most closely with the classroom teacher regarding the implementation of the Individualized Educational Plan (IEP).

The suggestion that one of these professionals function as the case coordinator does not imply a superior role for that professional. In the schools, this distinction rests with the clasroom teacher, who bears the greatest educational burden for all the children enrolled in the class, "special" needs or no. Indeed, the efforts of the case coordinator, and perhaps of all the "supportive" and administrative personnel in a school as well, make the most sense, in our judgment, when viewed from the perspective of the clasroom teacher. The "pay-off" comes in the classroom and it is there that efforts should most of all be focused.

○ THERAPEUTIC OBJECTIVES

Public-Law 94–142 requires the completion of an Individualized Educational Plan (IEP) for all "special needs" children, which of course includes the population of hard of hearing children, who are the concern of this book. It seems to us that an entire educational industry, including new personnel, procedures, guidelines, workshops, manuals, meetings upon meetings, and so forth, has developed since the inception of this law. The purpose of the law is to mandate procedures intended to guarantee that each "special" child receives the most appropriate education in as "normal" an educational setting as possible. In our ever more bureaucratically oriented society, it is sometimes difficult to separate this primary purpose from the morass of procedures ostensibly designed to most efficiently realize it. In other words, we sometimes lose sight of or de-emphasize what our real objectives are when we attempt to conform to all the bureaucratic demands made upon us. Thus, it sometimes appears that the proper completion of a form in a proper time sequence and with all the necessary signatures has more importance for some IEP participants than the actual, observable performance of a child. Nothing we do has any meaning if we cannot demonstrate, in some convincing fashion, that our children are somehow better off as a result of all of our efforts.

This is the reason for the comprehensive performance evaluation that each hard of hearing child should receive. It is the reason why the evaluations must be readministered on a regular, periodic basis, to keep track of the child's growth or lack of it, in all the dimensions of interest. We are required to relate our intervention methods with the child's status on these dimensions. Were our efforts, in other words, responsible for improvement, or would it have taken place if we had done nothing? Given a child's progress on one or more performance indices, what standards are we to use in evaluating the child's status? This is not a trivial question, as we shall see.

There are really three standards we must use in evaluating a child's performance. No one of them is specifically "correct" to the exclusion of the others. Each has merit and purpose. However, we are not going to communicate a child's status very well if we do not make clear which standard we are using at any given time.

The first standard is to consider the child's performance in relation to himself, to his own status on the dimension of interest (speech, language, some educational or psycho-social area). The question to ask here is how much progress has the child made in some intervening period of time? Sometimes the results can be quantified in terms of months or years of growth, such as to point out that the child has moved from a score of 5 years 6 months on the Peabody Picture Vocabulary Test (PPVT), or some other similar quantifiable language test, to a score of 6 years 3 months in a period of one calendar year. Or grade equivalency scores, such as can be derived from academic achievement tests, can be compared over a given period of time. Sometimes the child's progress does not lend itself to easy quantification, such as when considering the complexity or quality of a child's language or his increased confidence and ability to engage in oral communication. Quantitative comparisons, in any dimension that lends themselves to such analysis, are the easiest to make and are very valuable. Qualitative comparisons, in dimensions that are not easily quantifiable, are more difficult to make, but are, nevertheless, equally valuable.

Teachers and therapists should not make the mistake of ignoring a dimension simply because there is no easy way in which it can be quantified. Periodic, detailed descriptions of a child's capabilities and capacities will provide the basis for evaluating the child's status on some nonquantifiable dimension. In many respects, a child's personal growth is the most important standard we can apply. Basically, we are asking this question: Considering this particular child's potential, is he making the kind of progress we would predict and hope for?

The second standard is less useful, but still valuable. In this standard, we must consider the child's progress in respect to his hearing-impaired peers. Because, for the most part, the children we are concerned with are not being educated in separate classes with other comparable youngsters, in order to make this comparison, we must look at the demographic data that apply to this population. The question we have to ask is, how does this child's status compare with a similar population of hard of hearing children? There are, unfortunately, very little data available on this population to enable us to make this kind of comparison (what is available will be reviewed in the next chapter). One fundamental reason for this is that the critical dimension of hearing loss—the reason why we are involved with these children in the first place—is rarely defined adequately in studies that focus on the performance of hard of hearing children.

What is sometimes useful in judging this second standard is to consider the data available from the Office of Demographic Studies at Gallaudet College regarding the status of hearing-impaired children who are enrolled in special educational settings. Many of the children whose results are reported through the Office of Demographic Studies are quite comparable, in hearing level at least, to hard of hearing children in regular educational settings. Thus, their performance (usually worse than the "mainstreamed" hard of hearing child) does provide some basis for comparing the status of a particular child. This kind of performance comparison can assist in placement decisions; a child may be doing quite poorly in comparison with his normal hearing peers, but yet much better than comparable children in a more restrictive educational setting. Obviously, both of these comparisons have to be considered in making placement decisions.

The last but most important standard that should be used in evaluating a child's overall school performance has already been alluded to. It is one that many teachers consider to be "unfairly" applied to a hearing-impaired child—namely, comparing a child's performance to his normally hearing peers. We do not see how we can avoid making this kind of comparison, particularly now that we stress educationally programing a "special" child in the least restrictive educational setting.

One frequently finds comments in the literature pertaining to hearing-impaired children to the effect that separate test and performance norms have to be developed for them, because they are a separate population and have to be considered on their own terms. This reasoning is specious for several reasons. The hearing-impaired population is anything but homogenous in the one dimension that distinguishes them from the normally hearing—their hearing loss. Considering a "norm" for a child with no measureable hearing as being the same as one for a child with a 50 dB loss in his better ear simply does not make sense. Lumping together all these children under one norm tends to lower the expected standard of achievement to some lowest common denominator.

We have, in our judgment, been maleducating these children for years. Taking their average performance as the norm that we must strive to attain means simply to enshrine our poor accomplishments of the past. It is not a question of being "fair" or "unfair," but only of recognizing a reality situation. How can we aspire to some measure of "normalcy" if we apply different standards to their expected achievements? How can we make educational placement decisions with no knowledge of how these hearing-impaired youngsters compare to their prospective normally hearing classmates?

The point we have been making is that all three standards are useful and all can be appropriately applied to a particular child. It is necessary, as we stated earlier, to specify the standard being applied for a particular circumstance. We have on many occasions asked teachers and speech-language pathologists to tell us how some child was doing, only to receive incomprehensible responses. For someone to say that a child was "doing well" tells us more about the teacher or clinician than about the child. "Doing well" can mean that the child is not a disruptive presence in the class, or that the teacher/clinician is applying some idiosyncratic standard; it does not tell us how the child compares to his normally hearing peers, or if a predicted level of personal performance in some area has been achieved. Often, when we are given this response by a teacher or clinician, we can almost hear at the same time the unspoken qualification in their mind, "for this kind of child." If a personal standard is applied, it should be so stated. It is, however, absolutely necessary also to compare a hard of hearing child's status to his normally hearing classmates; otherwise we are simply ignoring the reality situation confronting a child and doing the child a disservice.

In the next chapter the literature on the performance of hearing-impaired children is reviewed. We will attempt to place the application of these standards in perspective.

The focus of this book is the hard of hearing child in the regular schools. We have defined this child as one who has developed his primary communication mode via the auditory channel and primary avenue of communication is auditory-verbal. Thus, in terms of our definition, the hard of hearing child has more in common with the normally hearing than the deaf child. The key to meeting the therapeutic needs of hard of hearing children is appropriate auditory management, which includes the early provision of amplified sound in order to preclude the effects of auditory sensory deprivation. In addition, however, a comprehensive performance evaluation must be completed on each child. The results of the program serve as the basis for planning a specific program of therapy. The objectives of the therapy program, for these children who are in a mainstream setting, must include a basis for comparison with their normally hearing peers. Given appropriate therapeutic management, the hard of hearing child, in our view, has the best prognosis for improvement of any child who displays a communicative disorder.

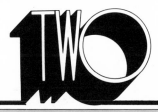

Performance of the hard of hearing child

○ CURRENT STATUS OF THE LITERATURE

Large-scale, published statistics on the performance of hard of hearing children in the regular schools are not available. There are fragments here and there, which we shall review in this chapter, but nothing at all comparable to the demographic data on hearing-impaired children in special educational programs published by the Office of Demographic Studies at Gallaudet College. The basic reason for this rather dismal lack is that hard of hearing children are not ordinarily enrolled in a special program (and when they are, it is probably because they have been managed or placed inappropriately) and thus are not easily accessible as a group for studies and evaluation. They are, rather, scattered in "mainstream" settings throughout the country, with no single public school administration, at any hierarchical level, able or interested in developing and collecting the information regarding their performance. This is an unfortunate situation, because such data would enable us to make relatively valid generalizations regarding their status along a number of performance dimensions and would enable us to compare their accomplishments as a function of any number of personal and management variables.

It would not be accurate to abstract, from studies dealing with hearing-impaired children in special educational settings, the data relating to children with lesser degrees of loss, and to consider such data as representative of the performance of fully mainstreamed hard of hearing children with similar degrees of losses. This would likely portray an overpessimistic view of their accomplishments and support a more, rather than less, restrictive educational placement for hard of hearing children.

Until, however, we are able to collect large-scale data on mainstreamed hard of hearing children, we will have to make do with the information we have available.

In all the dimensions of performance considered in this chapter, it would be well to keep in mind that for the most part research reports consider only the *average* results of a *given group* of children. Such data can assist us in understanding the general effect of a hearing loss upon a specific performance dimension, but cannot validly predict the effect of this sensory deficiency for a particular child. The difference between a general tendency and an individual's actual performance, between group and individual data, is an important distinction for the clinician/teacher to understand.

We will now review the available literature as it pertains to speech production, speech perception, language performance, academic achievement, performance related to degree of hearing loss, type of educational setting, and psycho-social status.

○ SPEECH PRODUCTION

A congenital hearing loss tends to produce speech problems; the more severe the hearing loss, the more deviant and less intelligible is the speech produced by the child (Montgomery 1967; Gold and Levitt 1975; Markides 1970; Monsen 1978; Boothroyd 1978). There are clear-cut differences between the speech of deaf and hard of hearing children, differences that appear more quantitative than qualitative. That is, hard of hearing children tend to make the same kinds of errors that deaf children do, but fewer of them (Gold and Levitt 1975), resembling in some of their productions the speech of much younger normally hearing children (Oller and Kelly 1974).

There appears to be a fairly good consensus in the literature regarding the nature of the speech errors made by hard of hearing children. Omissions of consonants, particularly in the word-final position, constitute about half the errors made (Gold and Levitt 1975). Accompanying the omission of the final consonant one can find the prolongation and nasalization of the preceding vowel. It is as if the child realizes that "something" is there, though he cannot accurately identify this "something," and he alters the preceding vowel in consequence of this imperfect perception. It is important to note that final consonants are either often unstressed or intrinsically weaker acoustically, and thus are not sufficiently salient to the hard of hearing child for him to easily hear such sounds.

As will be seen later, the child's perception of speech shows the same kinds of errors manifested in his production. Consonants using tongue-tip placement, as well as fricatives and affricatives, are more likely to be omitted than are other consonants. Hard of hearing children are also prone to omit one component of an affricate—for example, uttering /t/ for /ts/—or to distort the phoneme entirely. Here also, as with their frequent errors on the final consonants in words, their production errors appear to reflect and be a consequence of similar errors in speech perception (reviewed below).

Other speech problems manifested by some hard of hearing children include voice/voiceless confusions, and errors on compound and abutting consonants (DiCarlo 1968). When vowel errors are made, they are usually confused with vowels in close proximity in the vowel quadrilateral—that is, the vowel substitutions are usually correct in terms of frontness of the tongue but wrong in terms of tongue height or tensions. This placement, or tongue target error, is what often produces the almost, but not quite, accurate vowel production.

West and Weber (1973) performed a detailed phonological analysis of a four-year-old hard of hearing child, using the child's spontaneous language as material. Although the speech of only one child was examined in this study, it is possible, in our judgment, to make more valid generalizations applicable to the population of hard of hearing children by such a detailed analysis than by cursorily examining larger numbers of children. Therefore, the results will be discussed in some detail, in the expectation that other young hard of hearing children will tend to show similar patterns.

This 4-year-old girl had a 58 dB loss in the right ear and a 68 dB loss in the left ear (averages of the speech frequencies). Half the child's utterances were word-like and intelligible, and half were not. Even those that were not understood, however, were not babbling or jargon but linguistically structured units simply not understood by the examiners.

No consonant phoneme classes were uttered correctly 100% of the time in all contexts. Those that were fairly well established—that is, correct over 75% of the time—were /b/, /m/, /p/, /w/, /n/, /k/, and /h/. It will be noted that bilabials—that is, clearly visible sounds—predominate in this group. Another group of consonant phonemes was partially well established —that is correct more than 50% but less than 75% of the time. These were /d/, /ts/, /f/, /r/, /y/, /l/, and /t/. As can be noted, these phonemes require greater tongue-tip control than the previous phonemes, and thus are intrinsically more difficult. These are also phonemes that a normally hearing young child would tend to have more difficulty with, though their mastery of these phonemes would occur at a younger age than occurs with the hard of hearing child. This supports the notion that hard of hearing children are similar in their phonological development to younger normally hearing children. The last ten consonants were not established at all. These were /g/, /dʒ/, /v/, /ð/, /z/, /ʃ/, /ʒ/, /ng/, /s/, and /θ/. Most of these are also more difficult for the normally hearing child.

In summary, the child showed the expected pattern of development, moving from the ability to produce coarser contrasts in her speech to finer and finer ones.

We have been unable to locate any studies that included an analysis of the voice quality and prosodic aspects of hard of hearing children's speech. This is understandable; these children, as a group, probably do not manifest the kinds of deviations in these areas so clearly evident in the oral speech of deaf children. This conclusion is supported in a study by Whitehead and Jones (1976) that examined the duration of vowels in various consonant environments for normally hearing, hard of hearing, and deaf children. They found that the hard of hearing children modified their vowel durations in different consonant environments much more like normally hearing than like deaf children. They attribute the hard of hearing children's ability to make fine time distinctions in their speech to their use of audition in monitoring their own speech.

Such findings, in accordance with many others in other performance dimensions, lend support to the distinction made in Chapter One between deaf and hard of hearing children. The implication in terms of remediation is that speech therapy practiced with hard of hearing children can mainly be patterned on procedures followed with normally hearing children, provided the therapist can ensure the audibility and saliency of the phoneme in question with appropriate audiological management.

○ SPEECH PERCEPTION

The comprehension of a speech message entails more than the discrimination and identification of the acoustic components. In a conversational exchange, we do not ordinarily attend to the acoustic/phonetic features, nor indeed do we even consciously focus on the specific lexicon or grammar. We are, rather, concerned with meaning—that is, comprehending the message the speaker intends to convey to us. We accomplish this feat as economically as possible, in terms of how much informational detail we need to take from the utterance in order to understand the speaker (Booth-royd 1978). Normally hearing persons with a normal background of language development can often grasp the meaning of an utterance using only a fraction of all the potentially available information. They can bypass much of the acoustic, phonetic, lexical, and grammatical information contained in a speech signal because they share with the speaker much the same intuitive grasp of the language. Speaker and hearer share a learned, though usually unconscious, knowledge regarding the probabilities of phoneme sequence and occurrence, the grammatical and lexical constraints in any spoken message, and the rules underlying discourse as related to the situation and to the relative status of the participants (the pragmatics of spoken English). When listeners are faced with ambiguity, either acoustically or linguistically, they can delve as deeply as necessary into the message, right down to the basic acoustic/phonetic components, until the ambiguity is resolved.

For the normally hearing listener, then, speech perception is usually a global process, a search for meaning. Its prerequisite is a sharing of competency in the language of the speaker (Fry 1978). For the normally hearing individual, this competency is in general easily and effortlessly achieved through the sense of hearing, which includes the ability to auditorily discriminate and identify the acoustic/phonetic features of speech (Ling 1978).

The hard of hearing child is deficient in his ability to discriminate between similar acoustic elements, which consequently impairs his capacity to identify the acoustic/phonetic features of speech. Because of his impaired hearing, he is unable to develop the same competent and intuitive grasp of the language as do normally hearing persons. From the speech fragments he perceives, he cannot creatively reconstruct the intended message; he cannot, by means of a rich inner language matrix, synthesize the fragments into a meaningful message. He cannot employ his hearing to get to the global comprehension of messages without an extraordinary focus on the foundations of perception, the acoustic/phonetic elements of speech (Levitt 1978). The knowledge of a hard of hearing child's current ability to perceive these elements is therefore an essential preliminary to a rational program of auditory therapy. It is necessary to understand present status before we can move beyond it.

There is no question that hard of hearing children have difficulty in speech discrimination tests. There is an abundance of clinical reports to support this contention. What we have very little of, however, is controlled research that presents normative information or a detailed analysis of their speech discrimination abilities. Part of the reason for this is inherent in the usual conditions for administering these tests. Most congenitally hard of hearing children cannot be tested by conventional means, because of their deficient speech and language, and their inability to make written responses to speech stimuli.

It was precisely this problem that motivated the development of a Word Intelligibility by Picture Identification (WIPI) test for children (Ross and Lerman 1970). In one study using the WIPI test, twenty-one hard of hearing children, whose losses in the better ear ranged from 49 to 88 dB, achieved an average score of 59% (Ross et al. 1972). This is a closed-set response test in which the children select a picture from a matrix of six corresponding to the stimulus word. As such, a score of 59% cannot be considered to indicate good auditory functioning on the part of these children. It is, however, a fairly typical score of children who have not had a sustained auditory focus in their training.

A more analytical view of the speech perception abilities of young hard of hearing children was presented by Byers (1973). He evaluated the initial consonant intelligibility of twelve hard of hearing children, ranging in age from ten to sixteen years, with an average loss of 41 dB. With conventional speech discrimination measures (recorded W–22 monosyllabic word lists), the children achieved a mean score of 66%. Using the Fairbanks Rhyme Speech Discrimination test, Byers administered the test at five sensation levels (10, 15, 20, 30, and 40 dB above the speech reception threshold) and evaluated the children's responses as a function of the sensation level (SL). Starting at a low level of recognition at low SLs, the intelligibility of all stop consonants (p, b, t, k, g) tended to increase with increasing sensation level, with the poorest scores at all levels manifested by /p/ and /b/. The nasals /m/ and /n/ also showed poor scores at low SLs and an increase as the SLs increased, unlike the phonemes /r/ and /l/ and /w/, which showed a high score even at the low SLs. The children tended to show the poorest scores at all SLs with the /f/ phoneme, which is intrinsically one of the weakest phonemes in the English language. Surprisingly, considering its high frequency spectral composition, the children's performance of the /s/ was moderately good at all SLs.

Byers's study (1973) permits an analysis of the kinds of errors made by the children to the initial consonant stimuli. Table 2–1, adapted from his study, presents the confusions exhibited by the children (only the most common ones are included). Each number represents the percentage of responses to the phoneme stimuli. Thus, for example, on being presented with a /p/, the children responded correctly to a /p/ 41% of the time and incorrectly to /t/ 16%, to /k/ 15%, to /f/ 7%, to /s/ 8%, and to /h/ 7%.

As can be noted from Table 2–1, the most common errors made by the children dealt with place of articulation, while the features of voicing, manner, and nasality were usually retained. For example, the voiceless plosives were usually confused with one another, but rarely with a voiced sound (the original data show some minor exceptions); this is also true with the voiced plosives. Nasals tend to be confused with one another and seldom with other phonemes; the same finding is evident with the fricatives /s/ and /f/.

Boothroyd (1978), in his analysis of the speech perception capacities of hearing impaired children, also found that place of articulation is the pho-

TABLE 2–1

Percentage of Response to the Stimuli Phonemes for a
Group of Twelve Hard of Hearing Children

		P	T	K	F	S	H	M	N	B	D	G	W	R	L
	P	41	16	15	7	8	7								
	T	7	59	20		9									
	K	7	7	69		9									
	F	9	7		43	30									
STIMULUS	S				8	73									
	H		10	10	10	12	51								
	M							59	28						11
	N							13	79						
	B				10					48	22				
	D									12	69				
	G										8	78			
	W												63	28	
	R													81	
	L														73

Adapted from V. B. Byers 1973. "Initial Consonant Intelligibility by Hearing-impaired Children," *J. Speech Hear. Res.* 16, 48–55. Reprinted by permission.

netic feature most susceptible to the effects of a sensorineural hearing loss, while the perception of voicing, manner of articulation, and rhythm is perceptually available even to children with profound hearing losses.

Because there have been so few studies analyzing the speech perception capacities of hard of hearing children, it is necessary to consider the research on hard of hearing adults, in the expectation that some generalizations can be made that apply to hard of hearing children. Certainly, as was noted earlier, the entire process of speech perception for an adventitiously hard of hearing adult is not going to be the same as for a congenitally hard of hearing child. If, however, we restrict our consideration of adults to studies that have evaluated patterns of phonemic errors in restricted linguistic contexts (thus minimizing the contribution of the adult's linguistic superiority), then the task faced by an adult is not too dissimilar to that faced by a child. Such speech perception tests with adults focus on peripheral discrimination abilities—that is, the capacity of the impaired cochlea to differentiate between various acoustic signals having phonetic feature significance. This is also one of the initial stages faced by a congenitally hard of hearing child as he searches for the differentiating features in acoustic signals that he can incorporate in his developmental quest for language competency.

An important article by Owens (1978) summarizes the findings of a number of projects he and his colleagues have conducted over the years. In this article he reports on the results obtained with 550 sensorineural hearing-impaired adults who responded to the California Consonant Test, a closed-set speech discrimination test designed to elicit responses in either the initial (pin, thin, shin, kin) or final (leaf, leash, leap, leak) position. The subject hears one of the words, and responds by underlining the one he thinks he heard. The results reported by Owens with adults seem quite applicable to hard of hearing children as well. The probabilities are, in our judgment, that had a similar test been administered to hard of hearing children the same pattern of results would have been obtained. Even though, therefore, the Owens (1978) study concerns adults, we shall assume that the results also apply to children. Table 2–2, adapted from this study, gives the percentage of times errors could be expected for the different phonemes in the initial and the final position in words.

Some interesting generalities are evident in Table 2–2. First, the error percentages are greater in the final than in the initial position. It is more difficult to perceive the final sound in a word than the initial one, possibly because acoustically the final phoneme tends to be weaker than the same phoneme in the initial position.

Secondly, the magnitude of the error percentage is really quite significant. What these data indicate is that a subject, with no contextual cues, would err on the /s/ in the initial position 41% of the time and in the final position 53% of the time. As can be seen from the table, there are twenty-three phonemes where the error percentage exeeeds 25%, considering both the initial and final position. Inasmuch as these data were obtained with a multiple-choice response of four items, where chance alone would permit 25% correct answers, the magnitude of these errors is even more impressive (if that is the right word; perhaps the word "depressive" would more adequately describe the situation).

Finally, as Owens points out, if errors below 20% are disregarded, ten consonants are represented in both the initial and final positions—/p, t, k, tʃ, d , s, ʃ, θ, b, d/—and four in the final position only—/f, z, v, g/. Difficulties in consonant recognition, then, essentially reduce to these fourteen consonants (several others were omitted from the test because of the difficulty in developing suitable foils).

In addition to knowing what the error probabilities are for different consonants in the initial and final positions in words, it is important to understand the pattern of substitutions made when a phoneme is perceived incorrectly. Table 2–3 shows the most frequent consonant substitutions found by Owens and his colleagues. Substitution probabilities less than 10% have been omitted. The response substitutions are given in decreasing

TABLE 2–2

Error Probabilities of Phonemes in the Initial and Final Positions

The subjects were 550 sensorineural hearing-impaired adults listening to a closed response-set discrimination test

INITIAL STIMULUS	ERROR %	FINAL STIMULUS	ERROR %
s	41	s	53
p	40	p	51
k	38	z	47
d	35	k	46
θ	35	b	44
ʃ	33	t	42
b	33	f	41
t	29	θ	39
tʃ	26	tʃ	38
dʒ	26	dʒ	38
w	18	v	38
h	17	d	35
g	16	ʃ	31
f	15	g	22
v	11	n	11
l	8	l	5
r	6	m	5
		c	3
		r	0

Adapted from E. Owens 1978. "Consonant Errors and Remediation in Sensorineural Hearing Loss," *J. Speech Hear. Disord.* 43, 331–347. Reprinted by permission.

TABLE 2–3

The Consonant Errors Most Frequently Given in Response to the
Indicated Consonant Stimuli in the Initial and Final Positions

The substitution errors are listed in decreasing order of occurrence

INITIAL STIMULUS	RESPONSES	FINAL STIMULUS	RESPONSES
p	t k θ	p	t f k
t	p k	t	p k f
k	t p	k	t p
tʃ	t	tʃ	t k θ s
s	θ f ʃ t	s	θ f t p
ʃ	s tʃ	ʃ	f tʃ s
f	No percentages greater than 10%	f	p t s
θ	s	θ	p t k
b	v	b	ðd
d	b g	d	b v
		dʒ	d b v
		z	v d
		v	z d b

Adapted from E. Owens 1978. "Consonant Errors and Remediation in Sensori-neural Hearing Loss," *J. Speech Hear. Disord.* 43, 331–347. Reprinted by permission.

order of frequency; thus, for example, in the initial position for the stimulus /p/, the largest percentage of substitutions occurred with the consonant /t/, then /k/ and /θ/.

Comparing the data from Table 2–1, taken from Byers (1973), and the Owens (1978) initial consonant data (Table 2–3), more similarities than differences are apparent. Most of the substitution errors are made to consonants with different places of articulation. In the final position, however, more manner substitution errors took place than in the initial position (e.g., fricative substitutions for plosives and vice versa), though the predominant pattern of errors here too related to different places of articulation. Because previous data clearly pointed out that errors rarely cross the voice/voiceless boundary, and that nasals are seldom substituted for nonnasal sounds, possibilities for these kinds of substitutions were not included in the Owens (1978) study.

A few generalizations are possible. In respect to the pure-tone configuration and error probabilities, patients with configurations showing a sharp drop at 2000 Hz had difficulty with the /s/, the initial /t/ and /θ/, but not with /ʃ/, / tʃ / and /dʒ/. Difficulty with the latter group of phonemes occured only when the configuration showed a sharp drop at 1000 Hz. This observation accords very well with the data we have regarding the acoustic composition of the different groups of phonemes (Levitt 1978). The voiceless fricatives and the initial /t/ contain most of their acoustic energy above 2000 Hz, while the affricates still contain a significant amount of acoustic energy at 2000 Hz.

We want to reemphasize at this juncture that although much of the data presented in this section were obtained with adults, we can reasonably assume that they also apply to congenitally hard of hearing children to a large extent. In any event, because we do not have such data with children, we are constrained to make these kinds of assumptions until more specifically pertinent data become available. The clinical/educational implications of these findings will be discussed on a number of occasions in this book, beginning in the section immediately following.

auditory/visual perception of speech

We will not be reviewing in this book any studies dealing with the purely visual perception of speech for hard of hearing children. Such data are available or can be extracted from studies having other major purposes. Moreover, the focus on "lipreading" (or "speechreading") per se does not accord with the reality situation faced by hard of hearing children, and, indeed, such a focus may actually impede a rational therapeutic approach to these children.

The emphasis on speechreading for hard of hearing children appears to be a consequence of not making appropriate definitions and distinctions between the hard of hearing and the deaf child. In the oral education of the deaf, communication and language development through speechreading is an intrinsic component of the approach; without speechreading, there is no oralism. Because professionals made improper distinctions in practice between the hard of hearing and the deaf child, they tended to apply to the hard of hearing child a teaching method developed for the deaf child. The practice of scheduling hard of hearing children for speechreading lessons, then, by association with what was being practiced with deaf children, took on a great deal of credibility as a legitimate therapy approach.

In practice what happened, and what appears to be happening now, is that the focus of speechreading for these children is at the expense of capitalizing on their most efficient means of communication—their residual hearing. It is quite simple to devise "lesson plans" for speechreading; at the simplest level, one only has to drop one's voice while talking, using either unrelated nonsense syllables or words as stimuli (in which case, the therapist points out to the child the visual correlates of the speech stimuli), or using unrelated or related (through the external situation or the linguistic context) sentences. It is a great deal more difficult to ensure that residual hearing is being correctly exploited (see Chapter Three).

The emphasis on speechreading has tended to continue for a number of reasons, the most important of which seems to be sheer professional inertia (what is, tends to continue) poor training, background, and motivation. There is also another good reason, and that is that the term "speechreading" or "lipreading" had great public relations value. The public (and we include here administrators and parents) think they know what speechreading is. A therapist who "prescribes" a course of speechreading for a child gets figurative knowing nods from the public. The reasoning would be that this deaf child (has trouble hearing, therefore is "deaf") needs speechreading training. He cannot use his ears very well, so we must depend upon his unimpaired modality—vision.

There are several problems with this line of reasoning. First, we have no convincing evidence that we can teach children to speechread, beyond encouraging them to focus on the lips. Indeed, we have some evidence that the ability to speechread is related to the speed through which a visual sequence (the lip movements) is converted to neural messages and transmitted to the brain (Shepard 1977). In this study, a 0.93 correlation was found between the latency of a visually evoked response and speechreading ability for adults (it is a sad commentary on the continuity of research in this profession that this study has never been replicated, either with adults or, most importantly, hearing-impaired children).* Thus speechreading may be one of those faculties, among many others, for which human beings ordinarily show a wide range of innate capacities, and thus are not very amenable to training.

Secondly, the dependence of a hard of hearing child upon the visual aspects of a speech message varies according to the extent of his hearing loss as well as by the extent to which the speech utterance is masked by environmental noise. That is, the visual perceptual demands made on a particular child is a highly individualized matter, and cannot be met by a procedure that stresses soundless lip movements for all children as speechreading "therapy."

Finally, as was alluded to earlier, the stress on lipreading actually puts the emphasis on the less efficient modality in respect to developing and comprehending language. Audition, not vision, is the channel through which human beings most efficiently demonstrate their biologically determined ability to receive and generate the spoken word (Liberman et al. 1967). The corollary of placing a great emphasis on the visual by-products of the spoken word is that audition gets relegated to a supportive role, and that children exposed to such a program become primarily visual rather than auditory communicators.

We have no hesitation in recommending that visual cues (speechreading) be employed to enhance a hard of hearing child's total perception of speech. As a matter of fact, not only do we have no hesitation in making such a recommendation, we think it essential that these children use their eyes to complement the information they receive through their ears. There is a great deal of evidence to demonstrate that for the hard of hearing child,

*We have learned of one such study being conducted at the National Technical Institute of the Deaf in December 1980.

auditory/visual reception is clearly superior to that obtained by any single modality.

In a fairly comprehensive review, Erber (1974) reports on four studies showing that for the severely hearing-impaired child (whom we would define as hard of hearing) the mean advantage of auditory/visual perception over speechreading alone is 19% to 28%. In a different study (Ross et al. 1972), twenty-six hearing-impaired children obtained an average auditory word identification score of 52%, a visual word identification score of 48%, and a combined auditory/visual score of 68%.

More recently, Leckie (1979) has shown that even for very severely hearing-impaired children, with hearing losses greater than 95 dB in the better ear, when early and consistent auditory focus is applied in the children's training, the contribution of audition in an auditory/visual recognition task is significantly greater than that found in earlier studies on the topic (references in Erber 1974). She found an improvement of 23% for syllables alone, 33% for the final word in a low predictable sentence, and 36% in a high predictable sentence. Clearly these children were discerning the acoustic/phonetic characteristics of speech and not just the time-intensity pattern believed to be all they were capable of perceiving, in view of the degree of their hearing losses.

For hard of hearing children, it is important to make a distinction between unimodal or bimodal *recognition* scores and the *development* of language via a single or a combined sensory modality. The evidence, as reported above, is unambiguous as to the advantages accruing to the auditory/visual recognition of speech. But we do not know if language development can occur through, or is fostered by, such bisensory inputs. Indeed, there are some suggestions in the literature that simultaneous visual and auditory presentation may inhibit the learning of new material, and that when an apparent advantage occurs it is because the individual rapidly alternates between the two modalities and not because he processes them both at the same time (Gaeth 1967).

In response to this concern, and because of an emphasis on the potency of audition as the preeminent modality for language development, at least one well known teacher has stressed the initial training of hearing-impaired children only through the auditory modality, deliberately making visual clues unavailable for extended periods (Pollack 1970). Such an emphasis on audition is in accord with our personal educational philosophy.

As professionals, however, we should keep the question open regarding the possibility that language *development* can be fostered for some hearing-impaired children (including some with more severe hearing losses) with an auditory/visual approach, until at least more definitive evidence is available. The perceptual processes underlying bimodal reception, as will be discussed below, appear to support such a possibility for language development.

The analysis of speech perception errors made by hearing-impaired individuals demonstrates that most of their errors are due to difficulty in the auditory discrimination of consonants with different places, but similar manners, of articulation (Tables 2–1 and 2–3). Thus, for example, the /t/ and /k/ often are confused with /p/ (and vice versa); /b/ and /v/ with /d/ (and vice versa); and /θ/ and /f/ for the /s/. Rarely do auditory errors cross the voice/voiceless boundary in cognate phonemes (between the /t/ and /d/, for example), or are consonants with different manners of articulation confused often with one another (an /m/ for a /b/). When this and one other observation are combined, it seems to suggest that nature has provided us with an excellent opportunity to use vision and audition in a complementary fashion, one modality providing the cues not readily available in the other modality.

Consider the five homophenous (look-alike on the lips) groups identified by Binnie et al. (1974)—/p,b,m/; /f,v/; /ð,θ/, /ʃ,ʒ/; /t, n, s, z, k, g/—and their findings, supported in general by many other studies over the years, that *visual* recognition errors take place *within* and not *between* groups. On the other hand, *auditory* errors are rarely made *within* a group, because of the different manner and voicing features of the consonants comprising a group.

Almost perfect recognition, therefore is potentially possible when the visual and auditory cues are combined, at least for adults. The situation is not quite so promising for congenitally hard of hearing youngsters whose complementary use of different visual and auditory cues is of necessity tied to the status of their language competencies. That is, if such a child does not know the meaning of a word, he will hardly be able to recognize it even if all the elements are perceptually salient. This brings us back to the point made above, on which we do not have much evidence: Can such bimodal saliency underlie or improve the *development* as opposed to the *recognition* of language? The possibility certainly exists and should be considered.

In practice, hard of hearing children seem to depend upon vision only as much as is necessary for them to understand the message. When one presents to these children an optimal auditory signal, as would occur with an FM auditory training system, the children tend to keep their eyes on their books or their work, or if taking a test, on the paper. They soon discover that they can depend upon their auditory channel alone and do not require the additional information available through vision.

When using hearing aids in the same circumstances, however, with a distance of perhaps ten to twelve feet separating the speaker from the children, they tend to keep their eyes on the speaker as long as word or test stimuli are being presented; only when the speaker has finished do they bring their eyes back to the test paper. In this latter instance, the children soon discover that they require the visual cues in order to understand the message. This observation does not apply only to hard of hearing children; normally hearing individuals in a high noise environment must depend more and more on visual clues as the acoustic situation becomes progressively degraded through noise or other distortions (Sumby and Pollack 1954). Our task with hard of hearing children in regular schools is to maximize the auditory possibilities available to them, and only then encourage the complementary use of visual cues (but never as a substitute for good management of residual hearing).

○ LANGUAGE ABILITIES

vocabulary

When engaged in a face-to-face conversational exchange, many, if not most, hard of hearing children present very little apparent difficulty. They appear to have no problem in comprehending the speaker and in making appropriate responses. In such a situation, the child has a choice of vocabulary and language structures, and is able to select those with which he is familiar and which seem appropriate to the situation. This is true of all of us; we only tap a trifle of our language knowledge in any particular conversational exchange. If, however, one were to carry on an extended conversation with such children, particularly about topics removed from their experiences, and attend closely to the child's utterances, a less optimistic picture would begin to emerge. It would soon be noticed that the children seem to have much less flexible options in how they make a particular statement than do normally hearing children. The skilled listener would soon detect the presence of a number of pervasive language problems, one of the most important and underestimated of which is vocabulary.

Although the literature on the vocabulary status of hard of hearing children is not extensive, what studies there are are mutually supportive and accord very well with clinical impressions and experiences. Using the Ammons Full-Range Picture Vocabulary Test, Young and McConnel (1957) found that twenty hard of hearing children (mean loss 51 dB) performed significantly less well than twenty comparable children with normal hearing. Their finding that no hard of hearing child did better than any normally hearing child is particularly discouraging; we would hope that inasmuch as this study was conducted more than twenty years ago, when hearing aids were much less accepted than they are today, that this complete dichotomy of results would no longer be true. In our own experience, one usually finds *some* hard of hearing children performing better than *some* normally hearing child.

A more typical result of the comparable vocabulary status of hard of hearing and normally hearing children was given by Markides (1970). Also using the Ammons test, he found a two-to-three-year gap in hard of hearing children in vocabulary development (compared to four-to-five-years with deaf children).

Similar results regarding language status were found by Hamilton and Owrid (1974), with one interesting extension. They evaluated three groups of children, one with persistent conductive losses (average 32 dB), one with mild sensorineural (average 38 dB) and a normal hearing control group. Whereas the average vocabulary accomplishments of the hearing impaired groups was poorer than the normally hearing children (as expected), those children who came from higher socio-economic backgrounds did better than those hearing-impaired children from lower socio-economic backgrounds. Nonverbal test scores were the same for both groups. Superior results on the verbal tests also related to the reading habits of the parents: better reading habits, better scores.

The authors' conclusions were that the effects of hearing impairments are exacerbated in a negative socio-cultural background. One cannot completely ascribe these results to the fact that hearing aids are less available to the children from the poorer backgrounds; this study was conducted in Great Britain where hearing aids are given gratis to children under national health insurance. We would rather ascribe the results to a factor pertinent in any country: parental expectations and examples, and the consequences of these basically motivational factors upon a child's performance.

The vocabulary deficit of hard of hearing children is also evident in a study conducted by Davis (1974). She administered the Boehm Test of Basic Concepts to twenty-four hard of hearing children, who had losses ranging from 35 to 70 dB in their better ear. This test consists of fifty picture displays, which represent verbal concepts selected from basic kindergarten, first- and second-grade material. The test content includes vocabulary designed to assess a child's ability to identify space, time, quantity, and other miscellaneous concepts.

The Davis results show a decreasing ability of the hard of hearing children to recognize and respond appropriately to the test vocabulary as they got older. Of the 6-year-old hard of hearing children, 50% fell at about the 50% percentile, and the other 50% fell at or below the 10th percentile. Only 22% of the 7- and 8-year-olds scored at average levels, whereas 67% of the 7-year-olds, and 83% of the 8-year-olds scored at or below the 10 percentile. In other words, as the hard of hearing children got older, their vocabulary gap tended to increase. In Table 2–4 will be found the verbal concepts with which the children in the Davis (1974) study found the most difficulty. The numbers represent the percentages of children responding correctly to each of the concepts.

It is difficult to really get a "feel" for the vocabulary deficits exhibited by hard of hearing children only by looking at numbers, whether they represent percentages, chronological gap, or what have you. In our judgment, more

TABLE 2–4.

The Percentage of Hard of Hearing and Normally Hearing
Children Responding Correctly to the Indicated Verbal Concepts

	HARD OF HEARING	NORMAL HEARING
Not first or last	58	100
Right	58	87
Forward	58	100
Above	58	100
Widest	54	100
As many	54	93
Beginning	54	87
Third	50	93
Left	45	87
Few	45	87
Always	45	87
Skip	41	87
Equal	41	87
Between	37	100
Separated	33	100
Medium-sized	29	93
Least	25	100
Pair	20	73

Adapted from J. Davis 1974. "Performance of Young Hearing-impaired Children on a Test of Basic Concepts," *J. Speech Hear. Res.* 17, 342–351. Reprinted by permission.

significant vocabulary problems are ignored than addressed by this quantitative approach. A great deal of normal conversation at all ages is made up of idiomatic or metaphoric expressions, slang, and colloquialisms; in other words, any combination of words for which the meaning cannot be sought in a literal translation of the individual words. All hearing-impaired children (the deaf child more than the hard of hearing one) have a great deal of difficulty with combinations of words that do not literally convey their dictionary meanings. Such expressions change with age, with time, and with place, and the hard of hearing child has great difficulty "staying with it" or "moving with the flow."

Synonyms are another example of the kind of vocabulary that gives the hard of hearing child a great deal of trouble. He learns, or is taught, a single meaning for a word, or conversely just one word to express some general concept (for example, for bipedal locomotion, only using the word "walk," whereas, with a richer vocabulary, another individual could use the words "amble, creep, dawdle, stride, hike, trudge, ramble, march, tramp, traipse," and so on, to express nuances of meaning of the same concept).

In school, hard of hearing children frequently have trouble with specific kinds of academic tasks, not because they do not know the work, but because they simply do not understand the vocabulary (and sometimes the syntax) of the directions. The vocabulary contained in Table 2–4 is frequently included in the language of directions that children must follow in order for them to complete some academic task. Manifestly, this is going to be quite a feat for a child who does not understand the directions.

The child's problems, however, are not over even after the directions are explained to him (in simpler language, by example, pantomime, etc.); such children have an inordinate difficulty with the academic vocabulary, which begins to appear about the fourth or fifth grade. With normally hearing children, there is an underlying assumption that most of the new words are either already familiar to them or that there is sufficient linguistic context for them to comprehend the meaning. Neither of these assumptions necessarily holds for most hard of hearing children. Their vocabulary is largely based on speech directed (and explained) to them, in contexts with which they are familiar. They do not perceive or comprehend incidental language very well, that which flows around them in their home or school, or via television or radio; nor can many use linguistic context effectively to figure out the meaning of a new lexical item. The hard of hearing fifth-grader, suddenly being exposed in a science program to such language as photosynthesis, chlorophyll, ecology, producers, consumers, ecosystems, carnivore, omnivore, herbivore, and the like (taken from a fifth-grade science text), is simply lost and gets further behind as the years progress.

syntax

Superficially, there appears to be a great deal of literature available in this dimension of the language abilities of hearing-impaired children. However, a closer examination of this literature will reveal that almost all of it is concerned with children who are enrolled in special educational settings. Except for a very few studies, even those ostensibly devoted to hard of hearing children have drawn them from special programs, and thus cannot be considered representative of the much larger number of these children enrolled in regular school settings. From a research perspective, it is very convenient for an investigator to be able to draw their research population from a single source. Investigators, however, pay a penalty for this logistical convenience: their research results cannot be very easily generalized to the mainstreamed hard of hearing child.

The syntactical performance of hard of hearing children does not show the clear-cut differences from normally hearing children evident in deaf children (Quigley 1978). The differences observed in their syntactical performance appear to be differences in degree rather than in kind, with little difficulty shown by older hard of hearing children in the simpler syntactical constructions. This, as will be recalled, is the same impression one receives in evaluating the speech production development of hard of hearing children. The hearing loss appears to act as a depressant to the normal developmental growth pattern. Deviations, when they occur, are apparently due to insufficient and improper input at an appropriate developmental stage, with the child then using his linguistic rule-generating ability to create functional, though deviant, strategies for language comprehension and production. This interpretation is supported by the two studies we have been able to locate that specifically evaluate the linguistic abilities of hard of hearing children.

Wilcox and Tobin (1974) used a sentence repetition task to evaluate the verbal performance of eleven hard of hearing children, mean age 10 years, and mean hearing loss 61 dB. There were three experimental conditions: (1) repeating one of twelve sentences while looking at a picture depicting the event; (2) recalling a sentence after being shown the appropriate picture; and (3) repetition, where the child repeated the sentence without being shown the depicting picture. Using the third-person singular, the verb constructions selected for study were the present tense, auxiliary (be + ing), auxiliary (have + en), auxiliary (will), passive, and negative passive.

As expected, the results indicated that the hard of hearing children not only performed significantly more poorly than the normally hearing children, but also showed a much wider range of performance. Some of the hard of hearing children, in other words, did relatively very well, while others performed less well. None of the normally hearing children experienced much difficulty with any of the constructions. Of the six constructions evaluated, the hard of hearing children diverged most sharply in the cases of the auxiliary (have + en) and the negative passive.

The authors point out that in both these instances a word can be omitted without a resulting ungrammatical sentence. Thus, in case of the auxiliary (have + en) in the sentence "Mary has picked the flowers," the child can ignore the word "has" and interpret the sentence as a grammatical instance of a simple past tense. The same would be true in the negative passive sentence, "The glass was not dropped by Mary." In this example the "not" can be omitted, leaving a simple passive sentence in the past tense. In this latter construction, two simultaneous transformational rules occur, for passive and for past tense. Hard of hearing children apparently have a great deal of difficulty in applying two rules at the same time, as do normally hearing children at a younger age. A relatively small percent (16%) of the responses of the hard of hearing children were ungrammatical, which lends support to the delay rather than deviant hypothesis regarding the linguistic development of hard of hearing children.

The Davis and Blasdell (1975) study compared the performance of hard of hearing and normally hearing children in comprehending sentences containing medially embedded relative clauses. Their experimental subjects were twenty-three hard of hearing children, ranging in age from 6 to 9 years, with hearing losses ranging from 35 to 70 dB. The children listened to a sentence with an embedded medial clause and selected one of four associated pictures. An example of one of their stimulus sentences is, "The man who chased the sheep cut the grass." Additionally, they used the same surface structure to create sentences conveying different meanings, such as "The sheep that chased the man ate the grass." Again, as expected, the normally hearing children performed better than the hard of hearing children.

In support of the findings of Wilcox and Tobin (1974), Davis and Blasdell found that the normally hearing children made the same kind, though fewer, errors, than did the hard of hearing children. A greater range of scores was also observed with the hard of hearing children. The analysis of their responses showed that they adopted a processing strategy that shifted their attention toward the latter part of the sentence as the source of the underlying meaning. Thus, in the first example above, they would point to a picture of the man cutting the grass. Another strategy they used was to interpret the sentences in a contiguous fashion, using the closest subject, verb, and object sequence in processing for meaning. This latter observation also accords with the strategy used by young normally hearing children, who have the same difficulty processing embedded relative clauses as do older hard of hearing children. The responses of the hard of hearing children seemed much less certain; faced with an apparently confusing sentence, they would make responses that did not make semantic sense, but which they thought was required of them by the examiner. The hard of hearing children in this study misunderstood complex sentences 49% of the time. This is a very serious problem but not one usually manifested in social conversational utterances (how often do we use medial embedded phrases in our speech?).

The problem becomes evident when the child has to bring his deficient language skills to bear in his academic performance. Quigley (1974), for example, reports that relative clauses appear regularly in the second primer of a typical reading series used in the regular classrooms. As we shall see below, the difficulties hard of hearing children demonstrate in comprehending complex language (including vocabulary) is undoubtedly responsible for their typical pattern of deficient academic performance.

○ ACADEMIC ACHIEVEMENTS

Every study we have found that reports on the academic achievements of hard of hearing children, in mainstream or special settings, has shown that on the average the children are behind their normally hearing peers. It would be repetitious and serve no purpose simply to reveiw in detail all of the following studies (Steer et al. 1961; Kodman 1963; Quigley and Thomure 1968; Hine 1970; Hamp, Peckham et al. 1972; Paul and Young 1975; McClure 1977; Reich et al. 1977; Trybus and Karchmer 1977). There are, undoubtedly, other studies we have not found that report the same distressing circumstances. The situation, therefore, is quite clear and can be amply illustrated by simply reviewing only several representative studies. What may, perhaps, be more useful to the reader are some of the observations that can be made when these studies are reviewed carefully.

In 1963, Kodman reported on the educational status of 100 hard of hearing children enrolled in mainstream settings. The children were all in the normal range of intelligence and had hearing losses in the better ear between 20 and 65 dB. On the basis of their age, the children should have been placed in the sixth grade; however, their average placement was in the middle of the fourth grade. Inasmuch as these 100 children repeated on the average one and a half grades, this means about 150 extra grades repeated by just the children in this study. This is a common occurrence with hard of hearing children and, multiplied by the number of similar hard of hearing children in the entire country, represents a significant economic impact on this society (in addition to the personal cost of academic failure). Their average achievement scores were at the 3.8 grade level, which represents about two years academic retardation on the average. This two-year figure comes up time and again, and not just in studies completed many years ago, and can probably be considered an average deficit in situations where there is no or inadequate support services (Hine 1970; Hamp 1972). Of the 100 children in the Kodman (1963) study, only thirty-five were wearing hearing aids and only twenty-four received speech and language therapy. (In passing, and this will be elaborated later, it can be assumed that of the thirty-five children wearing hearing aids, only about a third of them wore functioning aids suitably adjusted electroacoustically.)

The same pattern of academic retardation can be seen in a study conducted five years after the Kodman study. In this study (Quigley and Thomure 1968), the academic performance of all the hearing-impaired children in Elgin, Illinois, was evaluated. Out of a group of 173 children, 116 were administered audiometric and IQ evaluations, and a number of subtests of the Stanford Achievement Tests. The age ranges of the students were fairly equally distributed, except for a sharp drop in the number of hearing-impaired children past the age of 15. The authors speculate that these children tend to drop out of school when they reach the legal age, probably because of the severity of their academic problems. (In our judgment, this is a very likely explanation and gives further support for the need for urgency in managing our hard of hearing children. When one considers, furthermore, that the percentage of hearing impairment is much greater among delinquent and prison populations than in the population at large, one wonders if the cost to society of mismanaging our hearing-impaired children does not extend much further than the academic areas.)

The results of the study were reported in terms of the hearing level of the better ear of the students. Several interesting findings emerge. First, there was a definite pattern of academic retardation, even for children with unilateral hearing losses (up to 14 dB loss in the better ear). They were behind an average of one year in word meaning, with the average of the various subtests (paragraph meaning and language) showing a deficit of about three-quarters of a year. The hearing loss category of 15 to 25 dB in the better ear showed an average subtest deficit of a little over a year, with each succeeding hearing loss category showing an additional gap of about a year, until the scores leveled off at about three years average academic retardation. The children at all hearing level categories performed more poorly in the word meaning subtest than in any of the others. This is basically a vocabulary test and the results support the previous comments regarding the severity of the vocabuly problems manifested by hard of hearing children.

The 116 children evaluated in this study also showed an average grade placement gap of a little more than a year, which, it will be recalled, was what Kodman (1963) found earlier. Only five children in the entire study wore hearing aids; if only the children in the more severe categories are considered (greater than 27 dB loss in the better ear), twenty of them were potential hearing aid candidates. This evidence for audiological mismanagement was mirrored in a similar lack of other support services.

We should like to reassure (if that is the correct word) residents of Elgin, Illinois, where this study was conducted, that they are not unique. Such evidence of inadequate management of hard of hearing children can probably still be found in the majority of communities in this country (and, no doubt, abroad as well).

Moving on to a more recent study, Paul and Young (1975) monitored the academic performance of fifty-eight children with mild to moderate sensorineural hearing losses (average at 1000 Hz was 40 dB) over a four-year period. The Metropolitan Achievement Test battery was administered four times during this period. A child was considered an "academic success" if his achievement scores increased by at least six months each academic year, with no more than a 1.5-year gap between his actual and expected grade level scores. More than a third of these children fall into the "failure" category (by this very lenient criteria). Additionally, because only the children's actual academic performance was considered, and not their ages, it is quite possible (even probable) that the results are yet more negative than they appear—that is, the children may well have been older than their normally hearing classmates.

A particularly discouraging facet of this study was the fact that half the teachers did not think that the children's academic problems had anything to do with their hearing losses, even though all of them knew the children had hearing problems. This finding illustrates the conflicts faced by a hard of hearing child, as discussed in Chapter One. Since he appears to "hear" and respond appropriately a great deal of the time, his teachers and other important individuals in his life develop certain normative predictions regarding his ability to communicate; when his responses become unpredictable, or when he appears to "tune out" or ignore a speaker, he then appears to be engaging in willfully negative behavior, for which he is penalized in one form or another. Such a child finds himself in a bind. On the one hand, because of his superficially normal appearance and communicative behavior, he is expected to act within a certain framework of expectations; on the other hand, because of his hearing loss, with the attendant language problems, it is impossible for him to do so. The encouraging aspect of the Paul and Young (1975) study was the program they developed to orient classroom teachers to the hard of hearing child. It proved effective in disspelling some of the myths and misinformation associated with the hard of hearing child.

In closing this section, we should like to point out that academic failure is not preordained. Children of normal intelligence do poorly academically because ineffective remedial measures are the rule rather than the exception. Although it is hardly realistic to expect that a moderate or severe hearing loss would have no effect upon a child's performance, we can reasonably expect to reduce the current prevalent academic lag displayed by these children. There are grounds for cautious optimism when we evaluate the products of good early management programs.

In one recent study (McClure 1977), fourteen mainstreamed children with moderate (56 to 70 dB) and severe (71 to 89 dB) hearing losses, who were the recipients of early amplification and auditory management, achieved average scores on the reading subtest of the Wide Range Achievement Test and low average scores in spelling and mathematics. The data were adjusted to levels of normally hearing children of the same age, rather than the same grade, and therefore took into consideration the fact that nine of the fourteen children had repeated one grade and were older than their classmates. The study by Reich et al. (1977) also showed a less severe academic lag than had been found previously with hard of hearing children, with the fully integrated hard of hearing child apparently functioning in reading and language at expected age levels.

Such studies are isolated examples of what could be, rather than of what is. There is no doubt that we can do better than we are doing. Professionals working with these children are in a fortunate situation; they can be assured that their devoted and intelligent efforts can really pay off in ways that they can see and appreciate (or as good positive reinforcement for the next hard of hearing child they work with).

○ RELATIONSHIP TO HEARING LOSS

Many professionals working with hearing-impaired children seem reluctant to accept the notion that a child's academic and communicative performance is related to the severity of a hearing loss. We have heard this reluctance expressed by very effective teachers, those who understand how to use a child's residual hearing to its fullest extent. Many of the children they work with function as if they had much less of a hearing loss, and therefore, compared to a child with a lesser degree of loss but whose performance is poorer, the degree of hearing loss appears to be a relatively unimportant consideration.

Although we do not doubt the excellent results that can be obtained with early and appropriate training, for the child with a severe to profound loss —indeed we have seen many such children ourselves—it does not follow that the degree of hearing loss is unimportant or that it does not relate to performance. The same excellent management would do even more for the child with the lesser degree of loss. The literature on the subject is clear: most studies show a significant, but not perfect, relationship between performance and degree of loss. What we have in these studies, in our judgment, are the consequences of less than optimal management— consequences that portray the relatively undiluted impact of the hearing loss itself on achievements.

The intelligibility of a child's speech decreases as his loss becomes worse. This general relationship was further analyzed by Montgomery (1967), who identified the hearing level at 2000 Hz in the better ear as the most significant frequency underlying speech production intelligibility. The importance of 2000 Hz was corroborated by Boothroyd (in Stark 1974, p. 45) for a population of "deaf" students. Negative correlations in the order of 0.62, 0.68, and 0.71 between an average degree of loss and speech intelligibility were found by Markides (1970), Jensema and Karchmer (1978), and Monsen (1978), respectively.

A number of investigators on this topic have pointed out that, whereas a good audiogram is a reliable predictor of intelligible speech, a "bad" audiogram does not always predict good or poor speech (Monsen 1978; Stark 1974, pp. 41–55). Obviously, as was alluded to earlier, a lesser degree of loss permits some natural development of speech, whereas the child with a more severe loss requires explicit assistance in using his residual hearing to assist him in developing his speech. The importance for speech production of degree of hearing loss per se, however, is amply illustrated by the strength of these relationships. As would be expected, the same type of relationship exists between speech perception and the degree of loss (Stark 1974, pp. 52–57). Which is to say that the greater a hearing loss children have, the worse they hear and the greater its impact upon performance.

Not so obvious as the foregoing relationships are the ones between the degree of loss and academic language abilities. However, the evidence supporting this relationship is also quite clear and unambiguous. When the language or the academic skills of the deaf and hard of hearing child are compared, the hard of hearing child (with the lesser degree of loss) achieves higher scores (Brannon and Murry 1966; Brannon 1968; Hamp 1972). When the relationship is evaluated between these dimensions and the degree of hearing loss for hearing-impaired children in general, the children with the lesser degree of loss perform superiorly (Hine 1970; Schulze 1965; Pressnell 1973; Jensema 1975; Davis 1974; Ross 1976; Trybus and Karchmer 1977; Gemmill and John 1977).

Table 2-5, one of the reports of the Office of Demographic Studies (Jensema 1975), presents a comprehensive view of this relationship for 6,871 hearing-impaired children enrolled in special educational settings. The data are presented as age deviation scores, with a score of 1.00 placing a student in the 84th percentile, and a score of −1.00 placing the student in the 16th percentile of his age group. These statistics compare a particular hearing-impaired child to the average score obtained by other hearing-impaired children, and not to normally hearing children. Note the progression from better scores to poorer scores, as hearing loss increases, but particularly in reading comprehension and vocabulary. The influence of degree of loss is quite apparent in this table. Note too the relative wide standard deviations at each data point; this illustrates the wide diversity to be found among a group of hearing-impaired children. They cannot by any means be considered a homogeneous group.

Incidental data in the table are also interesting. Note that about half the children have losses less than 90 dB. These are the children who, in our judgment, could be better served in a less restrictive educational setting, and whose performance is probably reduced as a function of the more restrictive educational placement (although, to be fair, many of these children were undoubtedly placed in the special educational setting because of failure in the less restrictive setting).

Exactly the same pattern of results was observed in a demographic study conducted in British Columbia on 383 school-age hearing-impaired children (Rogers et al. 1978). Beginning with hearing losses of less than 44 dB, the children's vocabulary and reading comprehension scores declined as a function of hearing loss. In the Canadian study, no decline was observed in mathematics scores (computation, application, and concepts as a function of hearing loss). With regard to academic abilities, a hearing loss quite clearly has its greatest effect on areas requiring the greatest degree of language competencies.

In reviewing these relationships, we do not mean to imply that the degree of loss is the only variable impacting upon performance. Certainly there are many children with severe losses whose achievements are better than those of children with less severe losses. Children with hearing losses display the same range of attributes as do normally hearing children; these affect a hearing-impaired child much as they do a normally hearing child. The hearing-impaired child with a high intellectual potential, a resilient and gregarious personality, whose parents have come to terms with having a hearing-impared child and can direct their energies in a fruitful fashion, is not constrained by these group statistics. Ultimately, performance is an

TABLE 2-5

Relationship Between Degree of Loss and Academic Achievement

The data are presented in age deviation scores, with a score of 1.00 representing the 84th percentile, and a score of −1.00 the 16th percentile. These data compare hearing-impaired children to other hearing-impaired children, and not to normally hearing children

HEARING LOSS IN ISO dB	N	VOCABULARY		READING COMPREHENSION		MATH CONCEPTS		MATH COMPUTATION	
		Mean	S.D.	Mean	S.D.	Mean	S.D.	Mean	S.D.
Normal (<27 dB)	64	1.28	1.27	0.78	1.11	0.50	0.89	0.19	0.86
Mild (27 to 40 dB)	140	0.85	1.36	0.65	1.30	0.58	1.11	0.28	1.04
Moderate (41 to 55 dB)	367	0.59	1.10	0.51	1.16	0.39	0.98	0.24	0.92
Moderately Severe (56 to 70 dB)	775	0.22	1.06	0.18	1.11	0.16	1.02	0.08	1.02
Severe (71 to 90 dB)	1838	-0.03	0.94	0.02	0.97	-0.04	0.98	-0.02	0.98
Profound (> 90 dB)	3464	-0.16	0.88	-0.12	0.87	-0.09	0.94	-0.04	0.96
Unknown	223	0.14	1.08	0.00	1.07	0.11	1.08	-0.07	1.07
All Students	*6871*	*0.00*	*0.99*	*0.00*	*0.99*	*0.00*	*0.99*	*0.00*	*0.98*

From C. J. Jensema 1975. *The Relationship between Academic Achievement and the Demographic Characteristics of Hearing Impaired Children and Youth.* Office of Demographic Studies, Gallaudet College, Series R, No. 2.

individual, not a group, matter. A hearing loss is a constraint, not an insuperable obstacle.

○ EFFECT OF EDUCATIONAL SETTING ON PERFORMANCE

Special education in the United States received a severe challenge in 1975 with the passage of the landmark Education for All Handicapped Children Act, Public Law 94–142. One of the important educational emphases of this law requires that children be educated in the least possible restrictive educational setting. For hearing-impaired children, the most restrictive educational setting would be a residential school, and the least restrictive would be full enrollment in their local regular school. It is necessary to ask if there is any educational merit to this provision. Does enrollment in a local school bring more benefits than problems for the average hearing-impaired child? In this section, we shall draw on the literature pertaining to both deaf and hard of hearing children, in special and regular settings, in an attempt to isolate the influence of the educational setting itself on performance.

This is not a new issue on the educational scene. We have long noted that hearing-impaired children in regular schools speak more intelligibly and perform better on language and academic achievement tests than hearing-impaired children in more restrictive educational settings. However, as has been pointed out repeatedly (Jensema 1975; Jensema et al 1978; Jensema and Trybus 1978), hearing-impaired children in regular and special schools differ on a number of demographic variables. The superior performance, therefore, noted for the hearing-impaired children in the regular schools may simply be a reflection of these other variables rather than of the educational placement. Other preselection factors may be operative as well. It very well may be that the children are in regular schools *because* of their superior performance, which antedated their educational placement, and that it is this initial status that is responsible for their later superiority.

Although all these considerations are no doubt pertinent, the weight of the evidence, as will be reviewed below, suggests that, all other factors being equal, the educational setting itself can either stimulate or retard academic and communication accomplishments. We shall first consider educational placement as a function of hearing loss.

From a study conducted in 1973 (Ross 1976), a report was made on the levels of hearing and performance of children in various programs under the aegis of a single school for the deaf. It was found that the children in the self-contained classes had an average loss of 97 dB, those in resource rooms in regular schools had an average loss of 83 dB, and those who were followed on the full integration program had losses averaging 76 dB. Although the children were assigned to the different programs on the basis of their academic and communicative functioning and not of their hearing loss, it turned out (as we would expect) that the children's superior performance was associated with lesser degrees of loss. All other dimensions of measured performance (word discrimination, bisensory word discrimination, PPVT, the preschool language scale, speech production intelligibility tests, and academic achievements) followed this same order: performance was better for the children in least restrictive settings.

Much more extensive data documenting this same observation were collected as part of the Office of Demographic Studies efforts (Jensema et al. 1978). This sample took in 945 children drawn from programs all over the country. The results are given in Table 2–6. Looking across the top row (residential school, residential students), one sees that only 7.2% of the students have losses of 70 dB or less, 27.5% have losses from 71 to 90 dB, and 65.3% have losses of 91 dB or more. In the lowest row (all part-time services, which includes fully integrated students), the trend is completely reversed. In this row 57.3% have losses of less than 70 dB, 24.2% have losses between 71 and 90 dB, and only 18.5% have losses greater than 91 dB. The in-between program types show the expected gradations between the extremes. Similar results were reported by Reich et al. (1977), who found that children in a fully integrated setting had more hearing than children enrolled in special programs.

The observation that children with less severe degrees of loss are enrolled in less restrictive educational settings is exactly what one would expect; making too much of this point is exactly the kind of pseudo scholarship that unfortunately too often passes as educational research. It is much more pertinent to ask, as was done earlier, whether enrollment in a less restrictive setting stimulates personal and educational advantages not possible in a more restrictive setting. There are some data that can be applied

TABLE 2–6

Program Placement by Degree of Loss

It will be noted that the less restrictive the program setting, the less the hearing loss of the children

TYPE OF PROGRAM	< 70 dB		71 to 90 dB		> 91 dB	
	N	%	N	%	N	%
Residential school Residential students	24	7.2	93	27.5	220	65.3
Residential school Day students	5	7.4	18	26.4	45	66.2
Day school	23	16.1	35	24.5	85	59.4
Full-time classes	73	26.7	85	31.1	115	42.1
All part-time services	71	57.3	30	24.2	23	18.5

Adapted from C. J. Jensema et al. 1978. *The Rated Speech Intelligibility of Hearing Impaired Children: Basic Relationships and a Detailed Analysis.* Office of Demographic Studies, Gallaudet College, Series R, No. 6.

to this question, and some legitimate—if one will excuse the phrase—commonsense speculations.

In the same Office of Demographic Studies report referred to earlier that plotted academic achievement as a function of hearing loss, Jensema (1975) also analyzed the effect of program placement upon academic achievement. As he points out, one would expect that children enrolled in different types of programs would be expected to perform differently (as they did), simply because of differences in their demographic attributes. However, even after correcting for some of the major demographic factors—such as degree of hearing loss—differences in academic achievement as a function of the type of program the children were enrolled in was clearly evident.

Table 2–7 was adapted from the Jensema (1975) study. The programs are organized from most restrictive on the top to the least restrictive on the bottom. We have modified the categories reported in the study, moving the "Resource Room" category between the "Full-time Special Educational Class" and the "Part-time Special Educational Class." This was done on the basis of the information given in the study, which suggests that the definition of "resource room" used results in an equally if not more restrictive educational setting than "Part-time Special Educational Classes." The category "Other" refers to children who are in regular classes full-time, receiving only that extra support available to other special children in the school.

As in Table 2–5, the results are reported as age-deviation scores, with the addition that the influence of certain key demographic variables has been eliminated. Note that the children enrolled in the top two categories (Residential School and Day School) are performing slightly below average for the hearing-impaired population, whereas the children in the Full-time Special Educational Class (located in a regular school setting) are at an average level. As the educational setting categories become less restrictive, the children's performance surpasses the average. These data strongly suggest that, other factors being equal, children enrolled in a less restrictive educational setting will outperform their peers in a more restrictive setting. The author of the study (Jensema 1975) remarks that other variables not accounted for may be responsible for the differences noted in Table 2–7, as indeed they may be. However, considering the important variables eliminated, the large population included, and the clear trend in the data, it is more likely that the results can be interpreted as given.

The salutary effect of replacement on performance was also found in a later report by the Office of Demographic Studies (Jensema et al. 1978). In this study, the speech intelligibility ratings of hearing-impaired children were related to a number of demographic variables, including degree of loss and program type. (In passing, we would like to point out that the ODS studies contain a wealth of important data on the status of the hearing-

TABLE 2-7

Age Deviation Scores in Four Areas of Academic Achievement as a Function of Educational Setting

The influence of degree of loss, age at onset of loss, number of additional handicapping conditions, presence of mental retardation, and reported ethnic background was corrected for in these data. In all areas of academic achievement, the children's performance tends to improve as the program type moves from the more to the least restrictive setting

TYPE OF SPECIAL EDUCATIONAL PROGRAM	N	VOCABULARY		READING COMPREHENSION		MATH CONCEPTS		MATH COMPUTATION	
		Mean	S.D.	Mean	S.D.	Mean	S.D.	Mean	S.D.
Residential school	3073	-0.09	0.82	-0.06	0.78	-0.10	0.84	-0.09	0.84
Day school	1018	-0.13	0.91	-0.14	0.82	-0.11	0.91	-0.11	0.86
Full-time special educational class	1975	0.04	0.90	-0.01	0.93	0.02	0.89	0.02	0.91
Resource room	192	0.19	1.07	0.22	0.97	0.17	0.93	0.13	0.92
Part-time special educational class	392	0.24	1.09	0.37	1.05	0.31	0.99	0.28	0.98
Itinerant program	215	0.69	1.23	0.71	1.20	0.56	1.02	0.42	0.94
Other	29	0.95	1.53	0.82	1.45	0.51	1.09	0.49	1.04

Adapted from C. J. Jensema 1975. *The Relationship between Academic Achievement and the Demographic Characteristics of Hearing Impaired Children and Youth.* Office of Demographic Studies, Gallaudet College, Series R, No. 2.

impaired child in special educational settings; the serious student in the field of deafness would do well to study them closely.)

Table 2–8, taken from their study, shows the relationship between the rated speech intelligibility of hearing-impaired children by program type and degree of loss. Note that for the students in the first column, with less than 70 dB loss in their better ear, the judged speech intelligibility was poorer for the students in the residential school, both day or residential, than for the students in the other categories. The converse is true in the last column, which shows the rated speech intelligibility of students with the most severe losses. More children in the day and integrated programs show better speech intelligibility than those in the residential schools (particularly for the residential students in the residential school.)

One could argue, as the authors of the study do, that within the less severe hearing loss category (less than 70 dB), more students in the residential school had the greater degree of loss, and thus it may have been the lesser degree of loss that was responsible for the better speech of students in the part-time services category. To a certain extent, this is probably a valid argument. However, it is not possible to make this argument for the children in the more severe category (more than 91 dB). In this category, the children in the less restrictive educational settings displayed better speech intelligibility ratings. In brief, the data strongly suggest that something is going on in the less restrictive settings, either to do with expectations, more experience with the normally hearing, or better speech and audiologic management, that fosters improved speech performance.

If these were the only studies reporting such findings, a cautious interpretation would certainly be in order, considering the implications of the findings for the education of the hearing-impaired child. There have been other reports, however, that corroborate the stimulatory effect of educa-

TABLE 2–8

Percentage of Students with Intelligible or Very Intelligible Speech (as Rated by Teacher) by Program Type and Degree of Loss

TYPE OF PROGRAM	< 71 dB %	71 to 90 dB %	> 91 dB %
Residential school Residential students	67	45	17
Residential school Day students	80	68	31
Day school	91	54	26
Full-time classes	85	62	24
All part-time services	90	51	39

Adapted from C. J. Jensema et al. 1978. *The Rated Speech Intelligibility of Hearing Impaired Children: Basic Relationships and a Detailed Analysis.* Office of Demographic Studies, Gallaudet College, Series R, No. 6.

tional placement performance. As part of a larger study, Hamp (1972) in England compared the achievements of eighty-seven hearing-impaired children in a residential program to fifty-three children with similar degrees of losses in a day school on a reading vocabulary test. The author found differences ranging from a half-year to almost a year in reading scores in favor of the day students. These differences were attributed to the higher standards and expectations existing in the day setting. The influence of the family was also considered (as rated by teachers) and found to be related positively to reading achievement, regardless of setting.

In an unpublished study conducted some years ago at the Willie Ross School for the Deaf, children who were in self-contained classes were compared to ten children who were fully integrated in their local schools. The children were matched as much as possible in regard to age and degree of loss. The results are given in Table 2–9. As noted, the two groups of children differ significantly on all the tests administered. Before we congratulate ourselves on the superior performance of the children in the "mainstream" setting, however, we should note that their accomplishments are nothing to be very pleased about. Although superior to their hearing-impaired peers in a self-contained setting, they are still far behind their normally hearing peers.

A much more extensive study was conducted in Canada by Reich et al. (1977). In this investigation, the authors assessed the academic, speech, and psycho-social status of hard of hearing children—on both the elementary and secondary levels—who were enrolled in different kinds of "mainstream" programs for different periods of time. At the elementary level, there was a total of 154 children, 77 who were fully integrated (average loss 42 dB), 42 who were also fully integrated but receiving extra services from an itinerant teacher of the deaf (average loss 54 dB), and 36 who were in special hard of hearing classes within the regular public schools (average

TABLE 2–9

Relative Performance of Two Groups (N = 10 in each group) of Hearing-impaired Children, One Group in Self-contained Classes for Hearing-impaired Children and One Group Enrolled in Their Local Public School

	SELF-CONTAINED	MAINSTREAMED
Age	8.6 yrs	8.5 yrs
PTA	82.1 dB	80.0 dB
PPVT	3.8 yrs	4.10 yrs*
Goldman/Fristoe	66.4	80.1*
Preschool Language Scale: Receptive	4.9 yrs	6.1 yrs**
Preschool Language Scale: Expressive	4.4 yrs	6.3 yrs**

*Significant beyond the 0.05 level

**Significant beyond the 0.01 level

loss 63 dB). There were 40 children enrolled in secondary schools, 12 of whom were fully integrated (average loss 41 dB), 17 also fully integrated but receiving services from an itinerant teacher of the deaf (average loss 47 dB), and 11 who were partially integrated, evidently in a resource room arrangement (average loss 69 dB).

The authors' findings both extend and corroborate the results of studies reviewed above. In academic performance (reading and language), the fully integrated children were performing at or above grade level, whereas the children receiving itinerant help or enrolled in special classes were a year or more behind their classmates. Of course, since the children's degree of hearing loss increased as their program became more restrictive, these findings are not surprising. The same pattern of decline was noted in speech intelligibility ratings.

More pertinent to our concern here, however, are the authors' (Reich et al. 1977) subsequent analyses and interpretation of their data. They reasoned that if integration is beneficial, then the children should demonstrate relatively more progress the longer they were enrolled in integrated programs. If, however, their superiority was the *cause* rather than the *result* of the integration, then the children who had been integrated for a shorter period of time should be performing as well as those who were integrated for a longer period (with other demographic variables equated as much as possible).

Their analysis suggests that the longer the children were in a regular program, the more their relative performance improved. This was also true for the children in the itinerant program, who progressed relatively more in language and speech the longer they were enrolled in the program. The setting itself, in other words, somehow acted as a stimulant (or a goad) for increased performance. Additionally, they found that the children in the hard of hearing classes fell further behind in reading the longer they remained in those classes. Similar trends occurred at the secondary level in academic and speech performance. One possible exception to this generally rosy picture occurred at the secondary level; the authors state that personal and social problems may be more severe for hard of hearing children in integrated educational settings. Although data in the study supporting this latter contention are, at best, tenuously suggestive, having some insight into the difficulties faced by such children in a regular school, we would certainly accept the authors' judgment as a general principle.

At about the same time, at the other end of Canada, another study was conducted, which, in addition to many other factors, also analyzed the academic performance of 383 hearing-impaired children as a function of their academic settings (Rogers et al. 1978). The settings the children were enrolled in ranged from regular schools, day classes in regular schools, classes in regular schools but administratively attached to a school for the deaf, classes on the campus of a school for the deaf, and special classes for problem children (no information is given as to whether the students in or attached to the school for the deaf were day or residential). In the analysis, the effect of the degree of hearing loss was statistically eliminated in the same way and for the same reason it was done in the Office of Demographic Studies reports: We expect the children in the least restrictive settings to display more residual hearing and we know that there is a high correlation between degree of loss and academic achievement. With the effect of degree of hearing loss eliminated from the study, the results in the two language related tasks (vocabulary and reading comprehension) show superior performance for the children in the regular school over those children enrolled in any other setting. The children in the most restrictive setting (classes on the campus of the school for the deaf) showed the worst performance in these two areas.

We have reviewed this issue at length because of its importance in the current educational scene. In our mind there is little doubt that, hearing loss and other demographic variables aside, the more fully "mainstreamed" the average hard of hearing child is, the greater his academic achievements. We can only speculate on the reasons for this phenomenon and apply some "common-sense" reasoning. In this field we are not often blessed with absolute certainty to support our judgments (though many of us too often act as if the "word" has been given us by divine intervention).

As one observes the children in self-contained classes, their own expectations and the standards of their teachers, quite clearly one sees a reduction in expected performance compared to normally hearing children of similar intelligence and background. The "norm" in a special class is derived, consciously or unconsciously, from the average performance of the children in this class. Almost always it seems much lower than what is possible. Until quite recently, most teachers of the deaf (although they are called teachers of the hearing-impaired and many also work with hard of hearing children) have had little contact in their training or experience with normally hearing children; moreover, many may not fully appreciate, because of inadequacies in their training, the potential of properly utilized residual hearing. Their efforts with the hard of hearing children in special classes are patterned after their experiences and expectations with deaf children. The children appear to be the victims of the dynamics of a self-fulfilling prophecy; by expecting their hard of hearing children to fall within the reduced level of performance manifested by the average deaf child, the teachers, not surprisingly, modify their standards in accordance with their expectations.

The situation is quite different for the hard of hearing child enrolled in a regular class with normally hearing children. The regular classroom teacher, not having much experience with such children, tends to expect from the hard of hearing child academic achievements within the range of accomplishments manifested by normally hearing children. When the "special" child, who appears otherwise bright and motivated, falls too far behind his classmates, the teacher is concerned and puts the pressure on. Or perhaps, the child, viewing what his classmates are doing, puts the pressure on himself. The parents also get involved and become concerned when the child's performance lags too far behind his normally hearing classmates. What we are saying here is that, paradoxically, those teachers who have *not* been trained to work with hearing-impaired children (both deaf and hard of hearing) may effect more positive changes in academic performance than those who have. We would hasten to add here, however, our other conviction that with appropriate assistance by such support personnel as the speech/language pathologist and the audiologist, and continuing orientation regarding the hard of hearing child, much more improvement in performance is possible with the average hard of hearing child than is currently the case. We should also like to add here the caution that these sentiments do not apply to the truly "deaf" child who, whether he is a candidate for limited mainstreaming or not, needs his special teachers and programs if the entire experience is not to be an unmitigated disaster for him. This book, we would remind the reader, is devoted to hard of hearing children; the situation with deaf children is included for perspective and because of frequent overlapping in educational placements.

○ PSYCHO-SOCIAL STATUS

One major problem in the behavior of hard of hearing children in a mainstream setting has been alluded to only briefly, and that is the psycho-social effects upon a child (Ross 1978). We would be remiss in our responsibilities to the children if we ignored such effects in our efforts to achieve the increased academic and communicative performance stimulated by integrated educational placement.

The older hard of hearing child, in particular, frequently feels somewhat like an outsider among his normally hearing classmates. Often he is the only hard of hearing child in his classroom or school. He may not know anyone else who has his handicap and, oddly enough, does not fully appreciate his own handicap (his very abnormality is "normal" for him). Many, particularly those who have not come through a good early management program, resent the fact that they have to wear a hearing aid. During adolescence, they may actively rebel against wearing an auditory training system or their hearing aids. Identity problems may occur; they neither hear as do other children nor are they deaf. No program dealing with hard of hearing children can afford to ignore their problems. They are not necessarily inevitable and they can be dealt with, as we shall see later; they dare not, however, be ignored.

Not only is there relatively very little research on the psycho-social status of hard of hearing children in regular schools, but what there is seems very inconclusive and contradictory. This is a very difficult area to research, with results heavily dependent upon such local conditions as availability of parent and teacher support programs, and the socio-economic and educational background of the children investigated. The studies reported do permit at least one cautiously optimistic generalization regarding the elementary school-age child: problems about social adjustment and self-concept are not inevitable (Elser 1959; Kennedy et al. 1976; Reich et al. 1977). The hard of hearing children reported in these studies are not indistinguishable from normally hearing children—differences do occur. The point is, at least as we evaluate the literature and our own experiences, that these differences appear to fall within an acceptable range of behaviors. This is not to deny the existence of problems, potential and existing, but to affirm that they can be alleviated or reduced with proper management.

Hard of hearing children appear to depend more upon the teacher for mediating classroom activities than do normally hearing children, who rely most heavily upon their peers (Kennedy et al. 1976). This is understandable when one considers the difficulty these children frequently have in following classroom discussions. As they get older, and become peer dominated (just like other "normal" adolescents), their personal and social problems may increase (Reich et al. 1977). As we warned earlier, however, these general tendencies can only serve as a backdrop to the situation as it exists for a particular child. His psycho-social adjustment is going to reflect a plethora of personal and social variables, and can be correctly assessed only on an individual basis. The solution, too, is going to be highly personal.

The point of all this is really to emphasize that whereas the hearing loss per se may increase the likelihood of negative psycho-social behaviors and adjustments, they are not preordained. Moreover, because the studies do deal with *group* descriptions, the ones we have seen on this topic seem almost irrelevant to the children as we know them. There does not yet seem to be an acceptable substitute for judging the psycho-social status of hard of hearing child than talking to him and his parents, asking about his friends and after-school activities and observing him in classrooms, cafeteria, and recess. We do not feel comfortable in making any further generalization regarding *the* psycho-social status of *the* hard of hearing child; there are just too many variations and not enough data.

In all the objective indices of speech, language, and academic performance, hard of hearing children seem to fall somewhere between the normally hearing and the deaf child. Their speech production and speech perception skills generally reflect the degree and configuration of their hearing loss, with place of articulation giving the greatest difficulty in both production and perception, while the manner and voicing dimensions (as well as the suprasegmental features) remain relatively unaffected. In their language abilities, the children appear to be delayed rather than deviant in their performance, giving results not unlike younger normally hearing children. On the average, academic achievements appear to be approximately two years delayed, somewhat less for mathematical computation skills and somewhat more for reading tasks. The degree of hearing loss is seen as a major factor relating to all performance dimensions, with more severe losses associated with poorer performance. The educational setting is also seen to be related to achievement scores, with the more restricted educational placement associated with poorer performance (even when the effect of hearing loss and other important demographic variables have been eliminated). Few generalizations can be made regarding the psycho-social status of hard of hearing children in the regular schools; while the effects of the hearing loss are a cause of concern and may affect psycho-social adjustment, the evidence suggests that this is neither widespread nor inevitable.

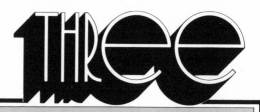

Evaluation of the hard of hearing child

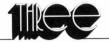

○ INTRODUCTION

No rational therapy plan can be developed for a hard of hearing child without a comprehensive assessment of his present status. In order to deal effectively with the problems which these children present, we must first understand them. However, it is also important to keep in mind that assessment is not an end in itself, that our responsibilities to a child do not end when we understand the nature of the problems he presents. This may seem to be an unnecessary stricture to insert at this point; we would like to assure the reader that this concern is based on real experience. We have often seen a hard of hearing child's problems described sensitively and comprehensively and yet noted that the child was still receiving inappropriate or insufficient therapy, with no real expectation of improving the situation in the near future.

In writing this chapter, we are assuming that the reader has had some introductory academic background in speech pathology and audiology. We shall not, therefore, review such basic content as the nature of various articulation, language, and audiometric tests, but rather focus on the application of these tools to the hard of hearing child. In the course of outlining a recommended test battery, we will comment regarding any modifications of the tests we have found useful, interpretations of the results, implications for treatment, and the need to disseminate and translate the findings to the appropriate individuals. In the sections covering the psychological and educational assessment of the child, we shall cover the material mainly from the perspective of audiologists and speech/language pathologists. We are not, it is important to note, assuming that we can do it all; the collaboration of our colleagues in psychology and education is a necessary ingredient in the comprehensive assessment of a hard of hearing child.

We can offer no set formula regarding the frequency with which evaluations should be conducted. At a minimum, we expect that each child should receive a speech, language, educational, and audiological evaluation at least once a year, with psychological evaluations conducted approximately every three years. Beyond this, the professional judgement of the individuals involved must be invoked concerning the need for more frequent assessment of any component of the comprehensive evaluation. The child should not be subjected to repeated evaluations to provide practice for a new therapist, or because it "would be interesting to know" the child's current performance on some specific dimension. Such repeated evaluations must have as their rationale clear-cut treatment implications, or they are simply a waste of everyone's time. With such treatment, however, where the results of the interim evaluations may carry important therapy or placement consequences, the clinician should not hesitate to schedule them. Audiological evaluations are frequently conducted more than once a year, particularly for the younger children, because of apparent shifts in a child's auditory functioning, or the need for modifications in the child's amplification requirements.

Although not covered in this book, the evaluation of a hard of hearing child cannot be considered complete until the requisite medical examinations have been conducted. This is often a continuing process, as it should be, particularly when the child demonstrates a progressive loss or recurring bouts of otitis media. At the same time, however, in addition to the purely medical considerations, a hearing loss carries with it important communicative and educational effects. The management of these latter factors should not wait until the medical treatment is completed, but in many instances may proceed simultaneously with such treatment. When managing young children with hearing losses, time is not on our side.

○ AUDIOLOGICAL EVALUATION

pure-tone tests

Since it is the hearing loss which is responsible for the child's problems, and indeed the reason why we are concerned with the child in the first place, an audiological evaluation is the first, and indispensable, component of a comprehensive assessment. Pure-tone air and bone conduction threshold testing begin the test battery. Perhaps because it is thought to be easy to administer, its value is often underrated. It is, however, the basic measure, the one which informs us about the type and degree of the child's hearing loss across frequency. It is administered either with a conventional hand raising technique or some form of play audiometry (Wilson and Walton 1978). Its apparent simplicity, however, can lead inexperienced or poorly trained examiners to commit such egregarious errors as overlooking a conductive component, over or underestimating hearing loss, or, in the case of a child with a pseudo hearing loss, requiring unnecessary medical treatment and/or amplification (Ross 1964). It is often necessary to modify the typical test procedures for younger children and for those with additional handicaps.* Thus its *apparent* simplicity does not imply an unskilled and untrained examiner.

*For further information regarding the young and difficult-to-test child, see Northern and Downs, 1978.

The information derived from properly administered pure-tone tests, both air and bone conduction measures, assists us in understanding the nature of the child's hearing loss and, at least generally, provides us with a general framework for relating the implications of the loss upon performance. Moreover, in spite of all the advances made in other types of audiometric tests, it is still the information gleaned from the pure-tone audiogram that carries the greatest weight for determining the specific amplification characteristics required by a child. We suggest that the air conduction thresholds of both ears be plotted in a chronological fashion, beginning with the first test which is considered reliable. This permits a longitudinal view of the child's air conduction threshold over time; observations of progression become clearly evident with this procedure. An example is given in Table 3–1 of chronological audiograms showing a progressive loss (for which a medical referral is required following a complete audiological evaluation).

As can be observed, only minimal shifts can be noted between subsequent tests in the early measures; it is only when the first three or four are plotted that the pattern of gradual progression becomes apparent. No conductive component was present as evidenced by bone conduction thresholds and impedance audiometry (not shown). Perhaps the dramatic shifts which occur later could have been precluded with an earlier medical referral, or maybe the nature of the educational recommendations would have been modified with this information. Even, however, if nothing would have changed with earlier knowledge, it is important for the professionals and the parents to understand the reality of the situation (genetic counseling comes to mind as one possible reason for having this information as soon as possible).

TABLE 3–1

Chronological Pure-Tone Air Conduction Thresholds of a Hearing-Impaired Youngster

No conductive component was evidenced by bone conduction thresholds or impedance audiometry.

DATE	RIGHT						LEFT					
	250	500	1000	2000	4000	8000	250	500	1000	2000	4000	8000
10/4/74	15	20	25	25	35	25	10	10	15	20	30	20
9/19/75	15	25	25	25	35	30	10	10	15	25	35	20
9/24/76	20	25	30	30	40	30	15	15	15	30	35	30
10/14/77	20	25	35	40	50	50	20	25	30	40	45	40
11/14/77	20	25	35	45	50	50	20	25	30	40	45	45
11/14/77	30	35	45	55	60	65	25	30	40	50	80	NR
10/8/78	30	35	45	55	60	NR	25	30	40	50	80	NR
12/8/78	35	40	50	70	75	NR	35	40	50	70	90	NR

speech audiometry

Speech audiometry is a necessary component of every audiological evaluation. Because the population we are dealing with is children, ranging in age from infancy (for exemplary public school programs) to high school or beyond, it is frequently necessary to modify the traditional procedures. Furthermore, because the primary purpose of these measures is to elucidate the communicative and educational situation rather than the medical situation (at least in our orientation), we further modify traditional procedures.

Speech reception thresholds (SRTs) are used to gain an overall estimate of the child's hearing loss and to check the validity of the pure tone thresholds. The SRT is defined as the lowest hearing level at which the child can understand 50% of the two-syllable spondaic words used as stimuli. The results are ordinarily highly correlated with the average pure-tone loss at 500, 1000, and 2000 Hz (the so-called speech frequencies), particularly in the two frequencies at which the hearing loss is least.

We have seen many children over the years who have failed hearing screenings in the schools, who have presented diminished pure-tone thresholds in the subsequent clinical evaluation, and whose pseudo hearing loss status was first suspected because of the discrepancy between the pure-tone and speech reception thresholds. "Pretending" to have a hearing loss, which is a less harsh and judgmental term than "malingering," is not an unusual occurrence with school-age children. Some children are prone to develop all kinds of ailments when having to go to school, or when a particularly unpleasant task (such as a test) is being scheduled. Children who have had some experience with hearing loss—either personally, with a transient middle ear condition, or vicariously, with a hearing-impaired family member—appear to prefer a hearing loss as their imaginary ailment.

The problem should not be minimized; it is important to know when a hearing loss is nonorganic. We have seen children scheduled for repeated and unnecessary otological examinations, fitted with hearing aids, and even undergo exploratory middle-ear surgery, because of pseudo hearing losses. Ruling out a nonorganic loss for children who fail public school hearing screening tests is one important reason why such children should be referred for a complete audiological examination prior to being seen by a physician.

SRTs also help us understand how well a child with a sloping pure-tone air conduction threshold configuration is using his residual hearing. If the SRTs of such a child agree much more closely with the pure-tone thresholds at the lower audiometric frequencies (250 and 500 Hz) than the middle and higher frequencies, we have some indication that he is making effective use of his residual hearing. If a child's speech or language status does not permit talk-back responses, it is acceptable and not at all inaccurate to use a picture or object pointing technique in measuring the SRTs. We also suggest that unaided sound field SRT's be obtained for the best overall estimate of the child's hearing loss.

There may be some children with whom an SRT cannot be obtained, because the ability to use their residual hearing is so poor—that is, they know that speech is being presented, but they cannot understand what words are being used. With such children it may be necessary to estimate their threshold for speech reception by obtaining a Speech Awareness Threshold (SAT). To obtain this measure the child merely has to indicate whether or not he has heard speech and not what he has heard. The SAT is approximately 10 dB better than the SRT and so a possible SRT can be predicted.

In the course of administering speech discrimination tests, the flexible and creative audiologist can obtain a great deal of useful information. The initial decision in such testing pertains to the specific type of test and procedure which is to be employed. In the conventional procedures, the tester reads a 50-word monosyllabic word list, presented in a carrier phrase, delivered at some constant sensation level (30, 35, or 40 dB SL above SRT), and requires the child to repeat all of the phonemes correctly. Some of the lists generally used with older children and adults are the PB-50 lists, W-22, Harvard lists, CNC, CVC, and others. For the younger child who is able to repeat back, the PB-K lists can be used (Appendix A). Such lists were designed to be within the vocabulary of kindergarten children and so are often more appropriate for the child with reduced vocabulary than adult oriented lists.

If the child's speech is quite deviant and his language and writing skills delayed and/or disordered, then conventional procedures cannot be employed and alternate methods are required, such as using the WIPI test (Word Intelligibility by Picture Identification), which is a closed-set, picture-pointing word identification measurement (Ross and Lerman 1970) with vocabulary at about the 3-year-old level. The scores on the WIPI test are typically about 20% higher than those which would be obtained on an open-set monosyllabic word list. In an extreme case, one child we saw obtained 80% on the WIPI test and 20% on a PB-K list. Such possible differences must be kept in mind when a closed-set picture pointing test is employed.

A number of precautions should be observed when using special or modified procedures. The following suggestions are variations of typical procedures which can be carried out in addition to regular testing in order to obtain more information about the hearing-impaired child. This information will be beneficial in setting up realistic goals for educational placement and all aspects of management.

(1) When possible, speech discrimination tests should be administered to both ears separately at an intensity level that approximates average speech intensity (about 40 to 50 dB hearing level, that is, dial reading on

the audiometer). If the severity of the child's loss precludes this relatively low intensity, then of course a higher suprathreshold level must be used—preferably at the child's most comfortable loudness (MCL) level.

The MCL is also an appropriate level to assess discrimination even when the child can be tested at a lower intensity. Obtaining discrimination measurements at MCL is based on the assumption that discrimination for speech is best at levels at which the child prefers to listen to speech. Some indication of the possible effects of amplified sound can be deduced by the difference between the discrimination scores obtained at a normal conversational level (50 dB HL), which may be insufficiently audible to a child, and at the MCL, which should, by definition, be sufficiently loud.

(2) Word speech discrimination tests should be scored for phoneme correctness rather than, or in addition to, simply marking a whole word right or wrong (Duffy 1967; Markides 1979). By analyzing the mistakes a child makes, it is possible to determine how well he is using his hearing, by comparing the errors to those expected from the configuration of the hearing loss. If the child cannot hear specific acoustic cues for speech, we cannot expect him to correctly perceive the phoneme that the cue distinguishes. For example, we can expect a child with a moderate high frequency loss to have difficulty auditorally distinguishing between phonemes with similar manners of articulation—for example, /f/ versus /s/, and the voiceless /th/—or to omit the weak final consonants in his responses. We do not expect such a child to confuse vowels, or consonants cognates—for example, /b/, /p/ and /m/.

Not only is a wider range of scores possible with phoneme scoring—for example, scoring the approximately 150 phonemes in a 50-word monosyllabic discrimination list—but the errors themselves become material for auditory management. For example, if a child cannot discriminate among the final /t/, /p/, or /k/, he can be alerted to the quality differences occurring in the vowel preceding these different consonants (the second formant transition of the vowels are characteristically different for these different consonants) and trained to make these perceptions. Another example illustrating the advantages of phoneme scoring would be where a child makes voiced/voiceless cognate errors in auditory discrimination (for example, confusing /t/ and /d/). There are a number of acoustic cues distinguishing cognate consonants (Levitt 1978) in addition to the simple presence or absence of voicing, which can be employed by a child in making such distinctions (see Chapter Three). In brief, this method of scoring is in keeping with our philosophy regarding the major purpose of the evaluation, which is that such tests must help clarify the direction and goals of management.

(3) As we shall see in the language evaluation of a hearing-impaired child, one must try to ensure that distortions in the speech perception process do not confound our efforts to measure the child's language status. This is a serious problem, and we shall spend some time discussing it later.

At this juncture, however, we are concerned with the reverse situation occurring—that is, where a child's deficient language capabilities are responsible for a reduced speech discrimination score. If a child does not know a word, whether it occurs in a closed set picture pointing test or an open-set monosyllabic word discrimination test, he is not very likely to get it right. Thus he may appear to demonstrate a more severe speech perception problem than he actually has, when the problem is really one of depressed vocabulary. When we examine the scores of such a test after the evaluation, however, we cannot easily separate out the relative impact of language. Consequently it must be taken into account when selecting the appropriateness of a particular test.

The development of PB-K lists or the WIPI picture pointing test, which use kindergarten vocabulary and a limited response matrix, was an attempt to circumvent this problem (Ross and Lerman 1970). When using the WIPI, for example, if a child makes an error the examiner can point to the correct picture and ask the child what it is. If the child does not know, it would appear that the stimulus item is not in his lexicon; if, on the other hand, he can correctly identify the picture, an assumption can be made that he did not perceive the item correctly, and the item would be scored as incorrect. However, the problem still remains that for a number of hearing-impaired children, many of the words on these tests (and all other language-based tests) are not known. Therefore, selection of appropriate vocabulary level items is not always possible, so errors occurring from language deficiencies must be considered during the evaluation.

Another way of controlling for language limitations, for those children who have basic phonic and orthographic skills, is to use a small number of nonsense syllables which the children have to point to or write down as they hear them. For example, present the syllables /ba/, /da/, /ga/, /pa/, /ta/, /ka/, /fa/, /va/, /cha/, /ma/, /na/, /tha/, /sa/, and so on. Different vowels can be used and the position of the consonant to be identified can be varied from the initial to the final position.

Such a test was developed by Levitt and his associates for use with deaf children and for comparative hearing aid evaluations (Levitt and Resnick 1977). It does offer the advantage of reducing the dependence on the subject's knowledge of the language inherent in conventional speech discrimination tests. Although such a nonsense syllable speech perception test has more face validity than a linguistically based test for hearing-impaired children, it appears to be used rarely, if at all, in the evaluation of hard of hearing children.

(4) The measurement of the child's most comfortable loudness level (MCL) and threshold of discomfort (TD) are simple, but valuable and often overlooked dimensions of hearing. At its simplest, speech stimuli are used rather than narrow-band noise or other acoustically more precise stimuli and both ears are tested separately. When measuring the MCL, the clinician

is trying to find the intensity level at which the child finds listening to speech most comfortable. It should be understood that the MCL is not a precise point, but a range, and that the instructions given by the examiner and the specific methods used to obtain it will tend to modify the results somewhat (Martin 1976, pp. 138–139). It is possible, however, to arrive at a moderately repeatable and valid estimate of MCL by alternately increasing and decreasing the level of speech (in essence, a modified method of limits) and asking the child for a most comfortable judgment.

We do not recommend the same procedure for the measurement of the TD. This can be a vital measurement, particularly if the selection of a hearing aid is involved (Ross and Tommassetti 1979) and we want to ensure that the child's threshold of discomfort is not exceeded when he wears a hearing aid. The child whose hearing aid delivers uncomfortably loud sound levels will either reduce the volume and thus not derive full benefit from the amplified sound, or reject the aid altogether. For the measurements of the TD, the speech level is slowly increased and the child is instructed to signal when it begins to be uncomfortable. The basic intent is to determine the highest intensity level which the child will tolerate.

It will be apparent to any audiologist who tests many children, particularly younger ones, that the measurement of the MCL and TD is more of a hope than a possibility. These are difficult judgments for younger children to make accurately, but should be attempted because of their importance. If these measures are not initially possible, they will be eventually as the child matures. The information they provide assists us in refining our knowledge regarding a child's auditory capabilities.

impedance measurements

In the relatively few years that middle ear impedance measures have been clinically feasible, a tremendously large and complicated body of literature has developed. In keeping with the assumptions we have made earlier regarding the probable (and recommended) background of the readers of this book, we shall restrict our comments on this topic to some pertinent suggestions and observations. In our judgement, impedance measurements must be included in every comprehensive audiological evaluation. Our hope, indeed, is that impedance measurements performed by an audiologist become included in the routine hearing screening now being conducted in most every school system in the country (Wilson and Walton 1978). We have already noted above the burgeoning literature concerning the educational and communicative implications of early and recurrent otitis media; impedance measurements are perhaps the most efficient way to detect and monitor the presence of this condition.

What is not so appreciated, perhaps, is that children with sensorineural hearing loss are also prone to develop middle ear problems, and that the effectiveness of their hearing aids and auditory trainers will be reduced when this condition occurs. In one personal example, we instituted monthly impedance measurements and otological examinations in a small school for the deaf. When we first started, approximately 40% of the children showed evidence of a conductive component, in one or both ears, superimposed upon their sensorineural condition, and were referred for medical treatment. After some months of this program, the incidence rate of a conductive component among the children was about 10%, indicating that the program was a success.

Impedance measurements are quick and easy to administer. The three measures are: tympanometry (determining the compliance—the opposite of stiffness—of the eardrum), static compliance (determining the volume of the middle ear cavity), and stapedial reflex thresholds (determining the sound pressure levels at which the stapedius muscle in the middle ear contracts). When making impedance measurements, a probe tip is placed in the external car canal. The tip has components which allows for the following:

(a) Introduction of a probe tone (typically 220 Hz). This tone may be transmitted to the middle ear via the eardrum, reflected back from the eardrum, or a combination of both. The amount of sound which is transmitted depends on the compliance of the drum; conversely, the amount of sound reflected back toward the probe depends upon the stiffness of the eardrum.

(b) Pick up of the reflected probe tone by a probe microphone. This information is relayed back to the impedance bridge and the compliance of the eardrum is determined by comparing the amount of energy reflected to the amount of energy transmitted. The stiffer the eardrum, the greater the amount of sound energy reflected back to the microphone probe.

(c) Air pressure in the external canal can be artificially changed (usually varying from +200 mm/H_2O to –300 mm/H_2O) by means of an air pump, which permits indirect measurement of the air pressure existing in the middle ear. It is known that the eardrum is most compliant when the air pressure in the middle ear equals the air pressure in the external canal. One can then determine the air pressure in the middle ear by varying the pressure in the external canal and finding the point at which the eardrum is most compliant (as determined by the amount of reflected sound energy).

The resulting tympanogram (air pressure along the horizontal axis and the relative compliance along the vertical axis) displays the relative compliance of the eardrum as a function of the air pressure existing in the middle ear. By comparing the obtained tympanograms to existing classifications (Martin 1981), the presence of different kinds of middle ear abnormalities may be noted (Figure 3–1).

The assessment of static compliance will corroborate the tympanometry results—that is the stiffness of the middle ear system can be determined by

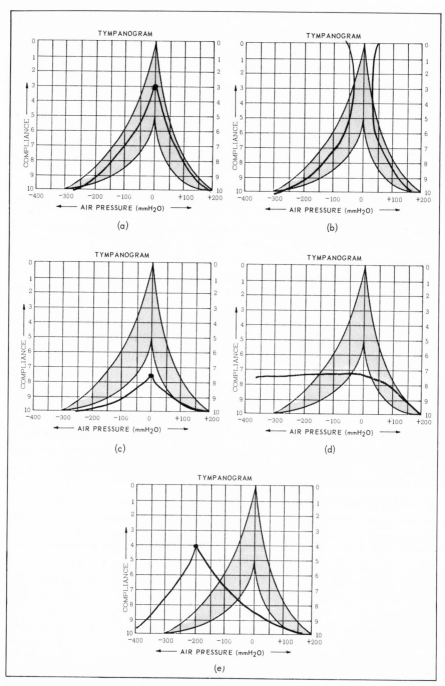

FIGURE 3–1a Tympanogram demonstrating normal tympanic membrane mobility and middle ear pressure, usually found with normal or sensorineural ears.

FIGURE 3–1b Type AD tympanogram demonstrating an extremely flaccid tympanic membrane, or an ossicular discontinuity.

measuring the volume of the middle ear cavity. The stiffer the middle ear (perhaps because of the presence of fluid), the smaller the measured volume. The normal range of static compliance is 0.33 to 1.66 cc. Any volume less than 0.33 cubic centimeters (cc) demonstrates an extremely stiff middle ear system. Any volume greater than 1.66 cc suggests a large middle ear cavity or perhaps patent ventilation tubes.

Stapedial reflex thresholds can reflect both the status of the middle and inner ears. When the stapedius muscle contracts (which it normally does reflexively to 70 to 90 dB SPL sounds), it tightens the ossicular chain, which in turn stiffens the eardrum. Since the stapedial reflex is bilateral, a loud sound introduced to one ear will cause the muscles to contract on both sides. Sound can be presented via a head phone to the nonprobe ear and the effects of the stapedial contraction will be observed in the probe ear— that is, the compliance will show a sudden change.

The inability to elicit a reflex within normal limits, or at all, could indicate that the sound was not loud enough,—there is a hearing loss—to get the stapedius muscle to contract. Absent reflexes can also be the result of some type of middle ear pathology, which frequently precludes the measurement of stapedial reflexes. Therefore, the absence of such measureable reflexes can indicate either a middle ear problem or a severe to profound sensorineural loss. The presence of elevated reflex levels are suggestive of either milder middle ear problems or a less severe sensorineural hearing loss. The presence of reflexes informs us that the child does not have a profound loss; the levels at which reflexes are obtained can be used as a guide for estimating the level of output at which a hearing aid or auditory trainer should be set (Ross and Tommassetti 1979). (All such measures can only be interpreted, however, in conjunction with other audiometric tests.) Figure 3–2 shows the results of an audiometric evaluation which includes impedance audiometry.

Impedance measures are particularly important for the child with a sensorineural hearing loss greater than 60 or 70 dB, because of the output limitations of the bone conduction oscillators above this point. Even children with a lesser degree of loss, for whom bone conduction thresholds can be measured, the difficulty in ensuring the appropriate level of masking still makes impedance measurement the test of choice for identifying the presence of a possible conductive component.

We recommend that impedance measurement be obtained on any hard

---

FIGURE 3–1c Type AS tympanogram demonstrating normal middle ear pressure but stiff tympanic membrane, usually found with otosclerosis.

FIGURE 3–1d Type B tympanogram demonstrating an extremely stiff middle ear system, usually found with middle ear effusion.

FIGURE 3–1e Type C tympanogram demonstrating abnormal middle ear air pressure, usually found with Eustachian tube dysfunction.

of hearing child who suddenly begins to show some behavioral changes, whether these are apparently auditory or not, even though it may not be time for the annual audiological evaluation. A child who begins to show disruptive behavior may be responding to a reduction in auditory information without knowing it himself.

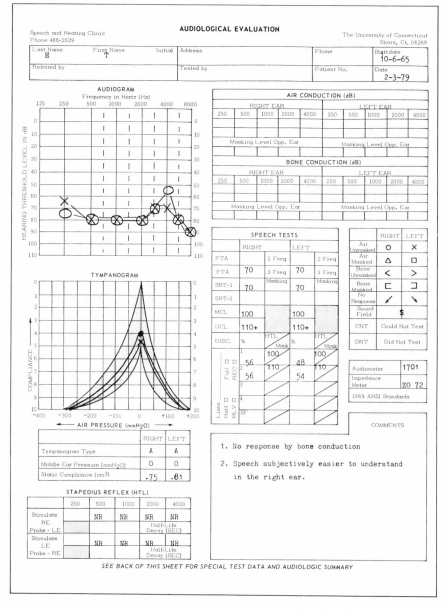

FIGURE 3–2 Complete audiological evaluation results, including impedance measurements.

We have also occasionally seen children who suddenly demonstrate an increase in acoustic feedback from their hearing aids, and are, therefore, unable to turn up the volume as high as they could previously, who upon examination have demonstrated a flat tympanogram typical of middle ear fluid. This result, indicating a relatively rigid eardrum, or a large amount of reflected energy, gave us the explanation for the increased "whistling" from the child's hearing aid. Due to the stiffness of the drum, the sound energy previously transmitted through the middle ear, was instead reflected back where it was picked up by the microphone of the hearing aid and reamplified, thus causing the feedback cycle.

Another change which would indicate possible middle ear problems is seen with children who make good use of their residual hearing to monitor their own speech. Such children may begin to show a deterioration in speech production intelligibility because of their deteriorating hearing ability.

○ AMPLIFICATION ASSESSMENT

If a child does not already use hearing aids, and he is a potential candidate, or if he has one and never used it, the first step of an amplification assessment is to remedy this situation. We have already expressed our conviction that the proper selection and use of an amplification system is the most effective therapy tool we have available. We simply cannot blithely go on with other therapeutic measures, expecting that somehow and someday, someone will supply a hearing aid for the child. We are the child's professional advocates, and even though we ruffle a few feathers by being pushy, we cannot tolerate delay; everyday a hard of hearing child is denied the benefits of amplified sound, he falls just a little further behind in the development of communication and educational skills.

In this section, we shall discuss the electroacoustic and behavioral evaluation of hearing aids and FM auditory trainers, which should be carried out at an annual audiological evaluation. Although it is a little bit of an arbitrary distinction, we shall defer the discussion of determining the need for a classroom FM auditory training system, and its proper and improper use in the clasrooms, until the chapter on management. The difficulty in making this distinction points out again the arbitrary nature of separating evaluation and management; in actual practice they are, and should be, mutually supportive and reciprocally dependent. (It seems that it is only when one writes textbooks that such an artificial distinction is made—probably because we are unable to create a more intelligent organization of the material.)

electroacoustic analysis

By electroacoustic analysis we mean measurement of the performance characteristics of the amplification system under carefully controlled and specified conditions of the physical environment—input sound pressure levels and so on—in accordance with the ANSI 1976 specifications. The purpose of the electroacoustic analysis is not basically to determine how suitable some hearing aid or FM system is for a particular child, though of course such inferences can be drawn from a number of the measurements, but to compare the unit's performance with the specifications as supplied by the manufacturer. Also, there are some dimensions of performance such as distortion which cannot be tested subjectively on a child, and it is only with an electroacoustic analysis that the clinician can obtain a precise insight into how the hearing aid is functioning.

The instrumentation to perform these analyses is becoming increasingly common in audiology clinics, and may also be found in some school based audiology programs. The instrument is basically a small soundproof box into which a loudspeaker is inserted. The hearing aid microphone is placed within the box and the receiver is connected to a 2 cc (approximating the dimensions of the average ear canal and middle ear) cavity which is coupled to a measuring microphone. The sound emitted from the loudspeaker is picked up by the hearing aid microphone, amplified and modified by the hearing aid, and delivered to the measuring microphone. This latter signal is then directed to some kind of response indicator, which displays essentially the difference between the input and output sound pressure levels.

Since amplification systems can be notoriously unreliable (Ross 1977), and since behavioral measures cannot assess such acoustic dimensions as distortion and compression characteristics, it is advised that an electroacoustic analysis be performed when (1) the aid is first delivered, and (2) at a minimum yearly interval thereafter. An electroacoustic analysis should also be scheduled when the behavioral and subjective measures suggest a possible problem.

We recommend that each child's folder contain cumulative results of the electroacoustic analyses, much like the child's audiogram, so that any differences that occur can be immediately apparent. Table 3–2 is an example of such a form. The gain (amount of amplification) figures can be obtained by subtracting the input SPL, usually 60 dB, from the output measures occurring in the basic frequency response curve. Half-octave frequencies have been included because of the valuable speech information contained at those frequencies. Some models of instrumentation used to measure the electroacoustic performance of aids may not record the same frequency figure noted in the table; in these instances, the clinician should select the closest frequency for recording (or construct their own form).

Each time a child's hearing aid or FM is analyzed, the figures should be plotted on the form and compared with the previous results. If all conditions of measurement are similar to those used previously, any modifications in the performance of the child's aid will immediately become apparent. Sometimes changes which occur may be positive, or at least not very negative, and such instances cannot justify changing a child's hearing aid. Sometimes,

Table 3–2

A Cumulative Record of a Hearing Aid's Electroacoustic Responses

Child's Name _____

Hearing Aid Make and Model _____ Date Obtained _____

Receiver _____ Tone Setting _____ Output Setting _____

Gain Setting _____ Output Settings _____

Date	Input SPL	GAIN											SSPL 90												Total Har. Dist.
		250	500	1000	1500	2000	3000	4000	6000	250	500	1000	1500	2000	3000	4000	6000								

Notes: (1) The frequencies listed may not accord with the preset frequencies included in hearing aid measuring equipment. Record the closest frequencies to those noted above.

(2) Gain is obtained by subtracting the input SPL (usually 60 dB) from the output recorded in a basic frequency response measure.

(3) The input SPL for output measures is assumed to be 90 dB in accordance with ANSI 1976 specifications.

(4) All conditions of measurement should be standardized as much as possible, e.g., input SPLs, tone and output settings, etc., so that this chronological record can truly reflect changes in the response of the hearing aid (or receiver pack of an FM unit).

however, glaring differences can be observed, which for one reason or another are not apparent in behavioral measures, and then the child should either have the aid repaired or receive a new one. For example total distortion figures should not exceed 10%; the maximum output (highest intensity the aid can produce at various frequencies) should not show a peak which exceeds the hard of hearing child's tolerance; neither should there be an excessive maximum output in the low frequencies compared to the middle and higher frequencies.

behavioral amplification analysis

Measuring the performance of a hearing aid or FM system, as it is worn by a child, provides us with the most valuable information we can obtain in estimating how suitable an aid is for a particular child. Certainly, such behavioral measures must be supplemented with electroacoustic analysis, but the final judgement regarding the appropriateness of a hearing aid or FM system can be made most validly only while it is actually worn by the child. Not only does the 2cc coupler used in electroacoustic analyses overestimate the physical dimensions of the ear canal in a child, but these coupler measurements do not include the changes in the acoustic signal that are created by earmolds, which can be quite substantial (Cox 1979).

In fact, the deliberate modifications of the acoustical characteristics of earmolds is one of the best tools audiologists have in refining the electroacoustic performance of a hearing aid. At the present time, their influence on performance can best be measured clinically by using sound field techniques, although this situation will hopefully change soon with the adoption and increased use of ear-canal microphones (Harford 1980). Earmold modifications can reduce low frequency response by venting the earmold; extend the low frequency response by extending the bore and narrowing its diameter; and extend the high frequency response by increasing the bore's diameter in a step-wise fashion, or by drilling a megaphone type cavity through the earmold; and the frequency response can be smoothed by the insertion of acoustical filters in the tubing leading to the earmold, or within the hearing aid tone hook. In short, to paraphrase an old cliché, the proof of a hearing aid is in the wearing.

A behavioral evaluation commences with unaided sound field measures. We have already noted the desirability of obtaining an unaided SRT, which gives the best estimate of overall hearing loss without amplification. If at all possible an unaided speech discrimination test should be administered at about 45 to 50 dB HL (this is possible only with children with no more than a moderate hearing loss). The scores obtained with this test enable us to judge how well a child would function at a normal conversational level without a hearing aid. These scores are later compared to those obtained at the same input level while using a hearing aid or FM auditory trainer and allow us to estimate the difference amplification systems make.

Unaided sound field tonal thresholds are also useful to plot. With proper calibration of the earphones and the sound field, it is possible to plot the unaided sound field thresholds by correcting the measured earphone thresholds (each ear separately) to arrive at equivalent sound field thresholds (Morgan, Dirks, and Bower 1979). However obtained—through correction of earphone tests or directly—unaided sound field measures are a necessary base on which to compare later results.

These same measures (aided warble tones, aided SRT, aided speech discrimination) are then repeated, this time with each hearing aid in place. *The primary purpose of the entire audiological evaluation is derived from this step.* From the information contained in the aided speech measures and aided warble tone audiogram, we can begin judging the suitability of a particular electroacoustic system (hearing aid or the receiver of an FM auditory trainer) for a particular child. Let us make this purpose explicit once again: we want to provide a hearing-impaired child with the greatest amount of the acoustic information contained in a speech signal consistent with the child's hearing loss.

In terms of an auditory training model, this is simply the detection level (Ling 1978), the other higher levels being discrimination, identification, and comprehension. We cannot predict what the child will do with this acoustic information; we do know, however, that the child's chances of maximizing his auditory potential will be considerably enhanced if he is given a richer supply of the acoustic raw material to work with (Fry 1978). Of course, some judgment of the child's ability to use the sound delivered to him can be derived from his aided speech discrimination scores. Given, however, the relatively crude state of current speech discrimination tests, we believe that a more refined estimate of the child's potential can be gained by considering the pattern of aided warble tone thresholds in conjunction with the known acoustic characteristics of speech.

In addition to the purely auditory presentation of a speech discrimination test, every hearing-impaired child should also receive a visual and a combined (visual/auditory) assessment. This test is usually done while the child observes the examiner through the test window. The purpose of this type of presentation is to try to determine the child's preferred avenue for sensory input, and to assess his ability to synthesize the visual and auditory aspects of speech. As was discussed earlier, the visual and auditory cues of speech stand in an almost complementary relationship with one another. In a three mode presentation procedure, using phoneme scoring for all modes, we can determine how well a child is able to capitalize on this phenomenon.

For example, consider a child with a moderate, bilateral gradually sloping sensorineural hearing loss. Listening binaurally in a sound field, he obtained an auditory alone speech discrimination score of 42%, a visual alone score of 64%, and a combined score of 88%. At first glance, the score of 88% in the combined mode would suggest that the child has little difficulty in comprehending speech, as is indeed true as long as he can see the speaker.

However, these results also indicate that he is not making sufficiently good use of his residual hearing; certainly, with a moderate loss (no more than 70 dB at 4000 Hz), he should be making better use of his hearing. In this instance, training therefore should focus on increasing his auditory capabilities.

In order to observe the effects of common acoustic conditions, this procedure can be carried out in the classroom in the presence of the teacher. The value of an FM system can also be demonstrated through a modification of this procedure (see Chapter Four).

In the next chapter, we shall illustrate the interaction between speech acoustics, the amplification characteristics of a hearing aid or FM system, and the child's hearing loss as plotted with a sound pressure level reference. Figures 3–3A and 3–3B are examples of a behavioral hearing aid assessment plotted in a conventional fashion.

communicating the results

In our judgment, a quantum leap in the audiological management of hearing-impaired children is attainable right now if audiologists would expend as much effort in ensuring the dissemination of their results and then the follow through of their recommendations as they do in devising and administering audiometric tests. If the persons involved in the day-to-day education of a child have not received or do not understand the implications of the audiological evaluation, or if they have simply ignored or overlooked the audiological report, we have been wasting a lot of time and money. More importantly, the very act of an evaluation raises expectations (which we often encourage): it carries with it an implicit promise that our expertise can make a difference in the child's life, else why the evaluation at all? We are accustomed in our society to having a diagnostic session, of any kind, followed by treatment. This continuity—diagnosis followed by treatment—is sundered in instances where the results and recommendations of an evaluation are not available or comprehendable to the individuals who are responsible for instituting the treatment.

We are not overly impressed with those who ascribe the communication breakdown, between the tests and their implications, to obtuse school authorities. In decoding our jargon, in explaining the communication/educational consequences of our findings, we have to meet them more than half way. In brief, our evaluation is not complete until we have expended every reasonable effort to ensure that our evaluation has some significance outside the clinic.

Writing an effective report, following it up with a personal visit and a personal explanation, and occasional phone calls, is more than the frosting on a diagnostic evaluation; on the contrary, such endeavors justify the entire procedure. The reports should go to all relevant personnel working with the child. It is also important for the parents to get a copy of the written report, not only so that they know what has been sent to the school, but so that they are kept informed as to the status of the child's hearing and amplification performance. This can help ensure their informed participa-

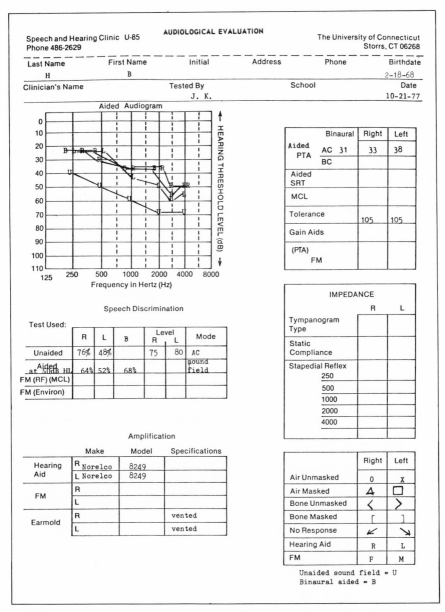

FIGURE 3–3A Hearing aid recheck results (on HB), indicating inappropriate high frequency amplification, as well as poor aided speech discrimination scores.

tion in the education of their child. Furthermore who has a better right
to be included?

Our communication with the parents must extend beyond this written
report, however. It can be devastating to a parent to receive a report which

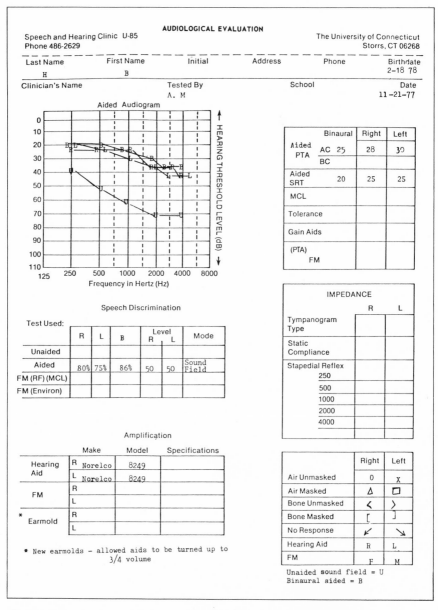

FIGURE 3–3B Hearing aid recheck results (on HB) after a new hearing aid had been purchased.
Note the improvement in the high frequency thresholds, as well as the aided speech discrimination
scores.

contains language with which they are unfamiliar. The audiologist is obligated to personally contact the parents and explain the results in language they can understand. The older child, too, should not be ignored. We have evaluated his ears and affected his life, so we should strive to explain his problem to him in ways he can absorb and accept.

The report of the initial evaluation is of necessity more comprehensive than the reports of follow-up evaluations. In the initial report, information is included regarding probable etiology (obtained from the child's physician), age of detection, all communicative behaviors (auditory responsiveness, speech and language status, gesture utilization), interpretive discussion of the audiometric results, initial counseling attempts with the parents (Luterman 1979), type of amplification system recommended, and provisions for an intensive follow-up in a parent/child program.

In this book, devoted to the school-aged child, we will assume that such an initial comprehensive evaluation has been completed (see Martin 1978, and Boothroyd 1982, for a complete account); our task here is to communicate the results of the continuing evaluations conducted for each child. Let us now consider the general components of such an interim audiological report.

(1) The first step is background—a review of changes in the child's overall status since the last evaluation. Have previous recommendations been implemented? If new aids, earmolds, classroom management schemes, or tutoring arrangements were recommended previously, were the suggestions followed? How is the child doing in school. Not just academically but socially? An interim evaluation must be considered part of a series, and subsequent assessments must be viewed as part of the continuity of management and not as an isolated entity.

(2) The presentation of the audiometric results usually follows the background. The type and degree of the child's loss is reported; any changes in any audiometric dimension are noted. If impedance measurements suggest the presence of a conductive element, a medical referral is required. Progression of loss also requires such a referral. The audiogram is explained in communicative terms in the report and personally to the parents, if they have accompanied the child, and then to the child in terms that can be understood.

(3) The status of the child's amplification system(s) is then reviewed. If he does not have one, or if a new aid is warranted, the audiologist presents the results of the hearing aid evaluation and reasons for the hearing aid recommendation. In the case of a child with mild to moderate loss, who has been "getting along" without an aid, the audiologist reviews the communicative and academic implications of the loss on the child and possible amelioration of these difficulties with amplification.

If the child already has a hearing aid, the electroacoustic data are presented (minus the technical jargon) and the behavioral results presented. The question to be answered here concerns the continuing appropriateness of this aid. Is it (or they) functioning as expected? Were electroacoustic changes made, perhaps to increase or decrease output or vary the frequency response; if so, what were they? Presumably they were made to increase the auditory potential of a child; how can such changes be expected to increase the child's reception of speech?

At this juncture, the audiologist is required to display his knowledge of speech acoustics. For example, as in Figure 3–3B, the audiologist should be able to communicate the hearing aid's influence on the child's increased ability to detect such high frequency phonemes as /s/ and /t/ and then communicate any implications of this improvement on the child's speech and language problems.

(4) Children outgrow their earmolds at fairly frequent intervals. If a new one is needed, either because of the sudden occurrence of feedback (but first consider the point made above regarding tympanometric results and feedback), or because it is desired to modify the acoustic properties of the mold, then this information is included in the report. In this instance, if the audiologist had taken ear impressions, the person or procedure for delivering the new earmold to the child must be specified.

(5) An evaluation report may include the necessity of a child obtaining an FM auditory trainer for classroom use. It is difficult—but not impossible —to make this determination just on the basis of a clinic-centered evaluation. Such a recommendation can best be made in cooperation with the speech-language pathologist as part of the continuing audiological management of a hearing-impaired child in the schools (see the section on audiological management). Depending upon the circumstances and location of the audiological evaluation, either a definite or tentative (to be corroborated by a personal visit in collaboration with the school personnel) recommendation for an FM auditory trainer can be included in the report. To reduce administrative confusion, we have found it helpful to write a separate report requesting such a unit for a child, because such systems are purchased by a school, unlike hearing aids, which are purchased by families or are obtained through other state agencies. (An example of a separate report requesting an FM system is given in Appendix B.)

(6) The final section of the report details and summarizes the recommendations made throughout the report. If new hearing aids, auditory trainers, or earmolds are required, this section should include all the details of these recommendations including adjustments—where they can be obtained, and reference to subsidary reports and contacts in respect to their acquisition. In other words, the report must specify how and by whom the recommendations will be implemented. The audiologist may want to comment on particular problems which should be considered in future evaluations. If there is a reason for a followup prior to the scheduled yearly evaluation, the date of the reevaluation should be included in the report.

In summary, the comprehensive audiological assessment should include:

1) routine pure tone and speech measurements and impedance; .
2) objective amplification evaluation:
    a) electroacoustic or listening evaluation of hearing aids
    b) electroacoustic or listening evaluation of FM
3) subjective amplification evaluation:
    a) speech discrimination and warble tone thresholds with hearing aids
    b) speech discrimination and warble tone thresholds with FM
4) report:
    a) updated background, audiometric results
    b) hearing aid–which settings, good volume, type of earmolds
    c) academic implications
    d) expected difficulties due to classroom acoustics
    e) recommendations

We can best demonstrate what was described in this section on audiological evaluation by example. Included below are representative reports on several hard of hearing children enrolled in the UConn Mainstream Project at the University of Connecticut. No one evaluation and the subsequent report includes all the evaluation components outlined above; moreover, because of the diversity of children and their needs, some considerations pertaining to these children may not have been discussed above. Both these points support the observation made much earlier—all these children have to be dealt with on their own terms and not in terms of some average concept.

case report #1

This report, taken from our files, concerns a 4-year-old child with a moderate, bilateral, sensorineural hearing loss. The referral information we received, which proved to be erroneous, indicated to us that he was going to be difficult to test. Firmly but kindly managed, he was quite cooperative during testing. He was also reported as having a tolerance problem, because he kept reducing the volume control on his hearing aids to the #1 setting. When the volume control was taped in place, and he was observed carefully, no tolerance problems were evident. This was possibly another method he used to manipulate his environment (everybody would pay a lot of attention to him when he turned the volume down). Since this report was written, an FM auditory training system was obtained for him.

Background Information JK was seen at this center for a complete audiological evaluation and hearing aid check on November 15, 1978, as part of the UConn Mainstream Project. J is presently enrolled in a preschool class at S School and was referred here by Mr. AM. J has a known bilateral moderate sensorineural hearing loss for which he wears binaural Zenith P5077 ear level hearing aids. He has been wearing the aids for approximately seven months and there is reportedly a question of tolerance problems because he turns them off. J has a history of middle ear infections, but Mrs. K reported that since his tonsillectomy and adenoidectomy in 1977, he has had no problems. This evaluation was to check J's hearing and amplification and to determine if tolerance problems exist.

Test Results Pure-tone thresholds indicated a bilateral moderate to severe sensorineural hearing loss. Speech Reception Thresholds (SRT) of 55 dB HL were obtained bilaterally, corroborating the pure-tone findings. Speech discrimination was 76% in the right ear and 80% in the left ear at 85 dB HL as measured by the Word Intelligibility by Picture Identification (WIPI).

Electroacoustic impedance measurements indicated normal tympanic membrane mobility, middle ear pressure and static compliance bilaterally. Stapedial reflexes were as expected (Figure 3–4).

A hearing aid check was performed with J's Zenith P5077 ear level hearing aids (¾ volume) in place. Warble tone sound field thresholds indicated that J was receiving appropriate gain from his hearing aids across the frequencies tested. A binaural aided speech discrimination score of 80% at 45 dB HL (normal conversational level) was obtained using the WIPI. It should be noted that no tolerance problems were observed at the maximum output of the audiometer when J was wearing his hearing aids (Figure 3–5).

An electroacoustic evaluation of the hearing aids was made using the Fonix 5500 analyzer. The aids are performing according to manufacturer's specifications with no significant distortion.

Impressions and Recommendations J continues to demonstrate a bilateral moderate sensorineural hearing loss. He appears to be obtaining good amplification from his hearing aids when they are set at ¾ volume. In order to keep J from turning the volume down, tape was placed over the volume control. It was also suggested that the volume control be marked with nail polish so that the correct level can be easily observed. It is recommended that:

(1) J use his hearing aids with the volume control taped at the appropriate setting.

(2) J use the available FM auditory trainer in school once it has been set for him.

(3) J return to this center for a check of his FM when he has worn it for several weeks.

(4) J have an annual audiological evaluation and amplification recheck to monitor the status of his hearing and his performance with personal and school-worn amplification.

I hope this information is of benefit to you. If there are any questions, please contact me.

case report #2

This report concerns an 11-year-old child with a bilateral severe to profound sensorineural hearing loss. He uses his hearing exceptionally

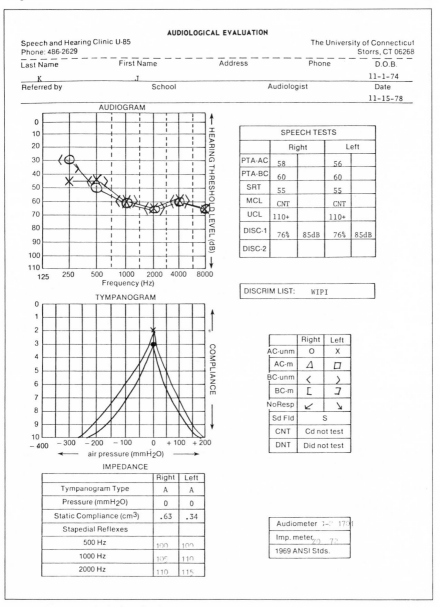

FIGURE 3–4 Audiological evaluation results for Case #1.

well, loves his hearing aids, and is doing well in school both academically and socially. Without the use of an FM wireless auditory trainer in
school, it is doubtful if his performance would have been as good as it
is.

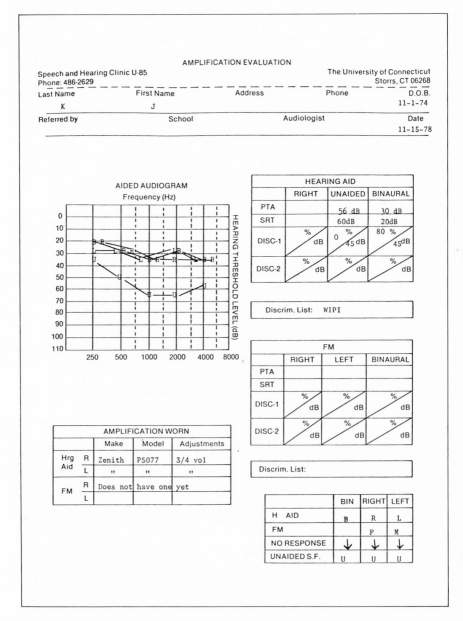

FIGURE 3–5 Amplification evaluation results for Case #1.

Background Information   L was seen at this center for a complete audiological evaluation on December 18, 1978, as part of the UConn Mainstream Project. L was referred here by Ms. FY, his speech-language clinician at H School. He has a known bilateral severe to profound sensorineural hearing loss for which he wears an Audiotone C401 body hearing aid (right) and a Zenith Heritage body hearing aid (left). Both hearing aids are approximately six years old and Mr. B expressed an interest in purchasing new aids for L. Today's evaluation was to assess the status of L's hearing and the functioning of his amplification systems.

Test Results   Pure tone air and bone conduction testing demonstrated a severe to profound sensorineural hearing loss with no measurable response above 2000 Hz in the right ear and a moderate to severe sensorineural hearing loss in the left ear. Speech Reception Thresholds (SRT) of 85 dB HL and 75 dB HL were found in the right and left ears respectively, corroborating the pure tone findings. Speech discrimination scores of 32% at 110 dB HL in the right ear and 84% at 105 dB HL in the left ear were obtained using the PB-K half lists.

Electroacoustic impedance measurements demonstrated normal tympanic membrane mobility, static compliance and middle ear pressure bilaterally. Stapedial reflexes were elevated (at 500 and 1000 Hz) or absent (2000 Hz), which is not unusual in light of L's hearing loss (Figure 3–6).

Sound field warble tone thresholds were obtained with L's hearing aids in place and were in a downward sloping configuration. These thresholds indicated that L was obtaining too much amplification in the low frequencies and not enough in the high frequencies. The binaural aided SRT was 25 dB HL and the aided speech discrimination score was 92% at 50 dB HL using the PB-K half lists. With L's Phonic Ear FM auditory trainer receiver in place, the aided sound field warble tone thresholds were 15 dB HL in the low frequencies extending to 55 dB in the higher frequencies. (Figure 3–7). At the time of the evaluation, the teacher's microphone was not transmitting, although it had been charged. L reported that it had not been working for "a while."

Electroacoustic evaluations of L's hearing aids and FM auditory trainer (environmental microphones) were made using a Fonix 5500 analyzer. The analysis of the hearing aids demonstrated that the Zenith aid was not providing enough gain in the high frequencies and too much gain in the low frequencies. The analysis of the Audiotone aid demonstrated that it was not providing enough gain in the high frequencies, was providing too much gain in the low frequencies and had more distortion than was tolerable. The analysis of the FM receiver unit demonstrated that it was not providing enough gain in the high frequencies, particularly in the left channel.

Impressions and Recommendations L continues to demonstrate a bilateral severe to profound sensorineural hearing loss. Based on the results of today's evaluation it is recommended that:

(1) L have a hearing aid evaluation to select new appropriate hearing aids.

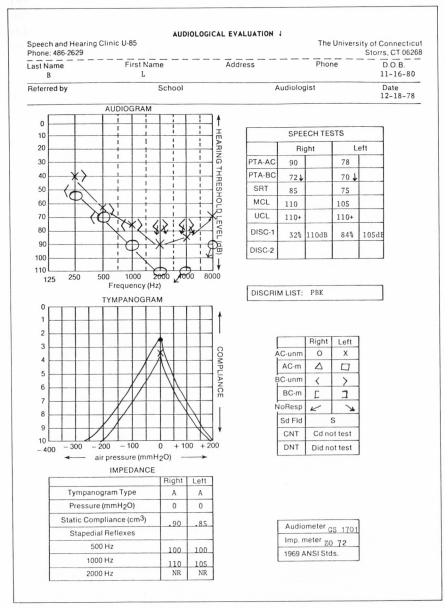

FIGURE 3–6 Audiological evaluation results for Case #2.

(2) The Phonic Ear unit be repaired and reset. The possibility of purchasing a new binaural unit which allows for separate setting of the channels should be considered. The importance of an appropriately functioning FM unit in the classroom to reduce the problems of noise, distance and reverberation cannot be overstated.

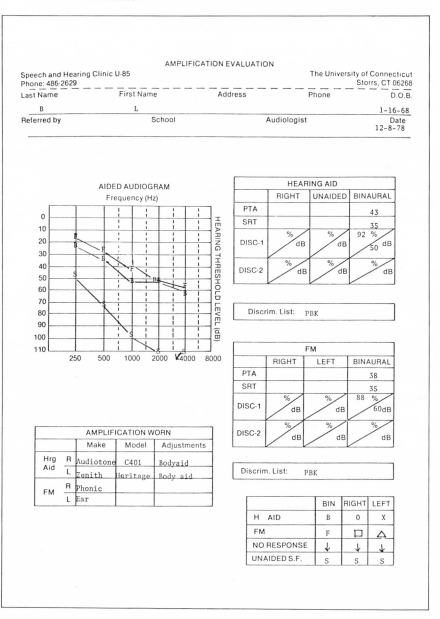

FIGURE 3–7 Amplification evaluation results for Case #2.

(3) L have an annual audiological evaluation to monitor the status of his hearing and amplification systems.

I hope this information is of benefit to you. If there are any questions, please contact me.

○ COMMUNICATION EVALUATION

Perhaps the weakest component of a comprehensive performance evaluation of the hard of hearing child is arriving at an accurate portrayal of the child's speech and language status. This is really a rather paradoxical situation; on the one hand, a hearing loss has its most dramatic effects upon communication abilities, but on the other hand, the tools for evaluating these abilities are among the weakest in the entire comprehensive battery of tests.

The profession has developed a number of tests for diagnosing speech and language problems in normally hearing children. Many of these communicative assessment tools can be employed with hearing-impaired children as well, provided the examiner is aware of the limitations and constraints in such circumstances.

Perhaps the major factor limiting the applicability of these tools for hearing-impaired children is the need to prevent the peripheral speech perception effects of a hearing loss from contaminating the results. In other words, when such a child responds incorrectly to a language based item, we must determine if the error truly reflects his language deviancies, or if it occurred because the message was distorted by a poorly functioning hearing aid, by environmental noise masking effects, or by inherent speech perception limitations.

If our intention is to evaluate a child's language knowledge—as determined by a standardized test—and he cannot accurately detect the acoustic/phonetic stimuli, the resulting score will reflect the impact of peripheral processing on his basic language knowledge. The influence of these contaminating factors represent the norm of the child's communicative functioning and provides us with valuable information regarding the child's functional ability. On the other hand, it is necessary to isolate, as much as possible, the effects of speech perception deviances from our language measures in order to develop an appropriate educational plan based on the child's specific strengths and weaknesses.

For example, in administering the Test of Auditory Comprehension of Language (TACL), we are attempting to measure a child's understanding of the morphological and syntactic rules of spoken English. If such a child makes an error with the plural marker /s/, is it because he did not hear it due to a poorly functioning hearing aid, the slope and degree of his hearing loss, the masking effects of noise, or is it because he does not understand the plural marking system? The same concern applies to the measurement of the child's comprehension of the grammatical marker for possession (Jeff's book), for the third person singular (he walks home), and for many contractions (it's for it is; let's for let us; and so on). The child's response to a test item is superficially similar regardless of the reason for his errors. But since the errors have different causes, the specific reason for the error must be ascertained in order to effectively plan a program of remediation. The same precaution is necessary when assessing all the unstressed morphological markers in English (e.g., /t/, /ed/, /s/, /z/, /d/, /ly/, /ing/, /ness/), particularly when they are of high-frequency spectral composition.

A similar careful analysis is required when assessing expressive language. The child may not be marking plurals, possessives, and contractions because of articulation problems, because he does not hear some of the unstressed sounds at the ends of words, or because he lacks the relevant linguistic knowledge. For a normally hearing child our communication evaluation tools can offer us only a modest glimpse into the child's underlying language competencies; for the hearing-impaired child, even this modest appraisal is not possible unless the complications wrought by the hearing loss are intelligently considered.

It is, therefore, frequently necessary to adapt the test presentation in order to more accurately measure a child's linguistic status. The stimuli may have to be presented several times, with the option of having the child imitate the examiner to ensure that he has heard the stimulus correctly. For some tests and for some children, written stimuli may be substituted for the oral presentation, or both oral and written stimuli may be used, and the resulting score analyzed for the occurrence of different errors in the different modes of presentation. All adaptations to a standardized test must be noted in order that the results be interpreted with the proper qualifications. This is particularly important for future reference when the same or similar tests may be employed to assess a child's language status.

Another major limitation of using conventional language tests with hard of hearing children is the relatively low age ceiling score of many of these tests. Once the older hard of hearing child exceeds this age, or reaches the ceiling score, we have no way of assessing his performance in a relatively standardized manner. Many older children have more or less obvious language deficiencies which cannot then be quantified, and thus their performance cannot be compared to other hearing-impaired or normally hearing children, or even to themselves over extended periods of time. This problem is beginning to be addressed with the influx of tests describing the language skills of adolescents. It remains to be seen how useful these assessment tools will be in describing the language competency of hearing-impaired adolescents.

It is doubtful that we will ever have standardized language measures which can accurately sample the awesome variety of normal language capacities in all its modalities (auditory receptive, oral expressive, reading, and writing), but certainly we can reasonably expect improvements in the present situation. The skilled examiner will, and should, have recourse to a careful, albeit nonstandardized, psycholinguistic analysis of the child's communication ability which allows the child to be compared with himself over time.

Such analyses require considerably more linguistic sophistication than is necessary in administering standardized tests. Readers interested in pursuing this topic are advised to examine the thoughtful and sophisticated analysis recommended by Kretschmer and Kretschmer (1978) in which a hearing-impaired child's written, signed, or spoken language sample is subjected to a semantic, syntactic, and pragmatic analysis. Leonard et al. (1978) also describe nonstandardized procedures for assessing a variety of communication skills, the specific content of which was taken from tasks used in psycholinguistic studies.

A fundamental purpose of analyzing a child's communication skills is to plan and administer an individually based therapy program. It is not, however, the only purpose of a communication evaluation. Mainstreamed hard of hearing children who are the focus of this book are expected to compete with and function alongside normally hearing children in their local schools. A hard of hearing child must be able to understand the content material presented in the classroom in order to follow the teacher's lessons and to participate in classroom discussions; he must be able to understand questions and produce intelligible and well-formulated responses; he must be able to communicate effectively, in and out of the classroom, both with teachers and other children. The results of the communication assessment must, therefore, be interpreted in regards to the total communication demands made upon the child in the school environment and then conveyed to all the school personnel who deal with the child.

The assessment battery we will be describing has been used by us not only to develop individual remedial programs and to monitor a child's progress, but also to help regular teachers and other school personnel gain insight into the communication problems of a hard of hearing child. Certainly, this battery does not include all, or even most, of the available tests on the market. The ones we will describe are included because they are accessible to most clinicians.

By considering the purpose of a communicative assessment, as we have noted above, it should be possible to evaluate the potential usefulness of any other possible test and add it to the battery if desirable. This battery of tests is not prescribed for all times and for all children. The battery we use changes each year as we eliminate some tests and include others; some tests are appropriate for some children and not for others, because of age differences and large variations in communication skills. We would caution the reader, however, that tests have no intrinsic merit divorced from their therapeutic application. It is only possible to justify the time children and clinicians spend in taking and administering these tests when their results are applied to improve the child's communication performance.

predominant mode for speech reception

We have found it very useful to provide teachers with a clear illustration of the child's capacity to receive speech through the visual and auditory channels, separately and in combination. This is accomplished in the school setting through either the speech language pathologist or the audiologist administering the PB-K word lists (see Appendix A) under three receiving conditions and having the child repeat what he perceives. The examiner administers one list without voice for the speech-reading condition, another one while covering the mouth for the auditory condition, and a third while the child can both see the examiner's lips and hear the stimuli.

By giving the tests in the regular classroom, while the other children are engaged in seat work or small group activities, the effect of noise and other classroom distractions upon the child's receptive capacities through the three modalities can be convincingly conveyed to the teacher. The procedure has the merit of evident face validity, and while it is no substitute for more controlled measures of speech discrimination in a clinic (also under the three modalities), the implications of the results can be easily explained to the child's teacher—who desirably is present during the test administration. With children for whom the PB-K lists are too difficult, either because of their age or language level, we use the Word Intelligibility by Picture Identification test (WIPI, Ross and Lerman 1970). The results are analyzed and discussed in terms of the child's predominant mode for speech reception with their implications for modifying classroom presentations.

We expect that the scores obtained in the combined look/listen mode will be higher than those observed in either single modality condition, confirming the complementary contribution of speech reading and audition in the speech reception scores of hard of hearing listeners (as reviewed in Chapter Two). Comparing the single modality scores enables the examiner to gain some insight into whether a child depends primarily on one or the other channel, or neither, and their relative contributions toward combined reception.

For example, consider two children with very similar hearing losses who both achieve combined reception scores of 84%. Superficially, it would appear that they are functioning in a comparable fashion. However, the single modality scores of the first child was 30% for speechreading and 62% for listening, while for the second child, the situation was reversed with the speechreading score being 60% and the listening score 32%. Such results can serve two definite purposes for clinicians: one concerning setting individual therapy goals, and the other for raising teacher sensitivity to a child's needs.

The first purpose concerns the disparity in the speechreading and listening scores between the two children. Considering their comparable hearing losses, and assuming that they are not too dissimilar in other respects, the clinician must seek to understand the reason for the disparity. Each modality makes a contribution to combined speech reception; if it is possible to enhance the functioning of the poorer modality, where clearly there is room for improvement, then the effect would be to increase combined modality reception. It is, in our judgment, easier to improve auditory scores than visual, through the application of the appropriate auditory management procedures (see Chapter Four).

The second purpose probably has the most immediate impact for hard of hearing children and their teachers. Many teachers then think that if the child is wearing a hearing aid then no further action is necessary on their part. They also think that if he can see the teacher's lips, the child can follow the classroom discussion and lessons just through speechreading. The improvement over single modalities wrought by combined reception is sometimes quite a revelation for them. After seeing such results, teachers are more willing to making modifications in their teaching style in order to maximize the child's reception of speech—such as not talking to the blackboard, or with a pencil jutting out of one corner of their mouths.

As we stated earlier, the in-classroom procedure is no substitute for controlled measurements of auditory discrimination (or speechreading and combined reception as well). Administered live-voice in a face to face fashion, the procedure is undoubtedly influenced by a number of variables which would affect the results. We do not use the scores in any absolute sense, but rather relatively, comparing the scores a single child achieves under the three modalities. This relative comparison enables us to make generalizations regarding a child's predominant mode of speech reception. The face validity of the procedure could be increased if sentence, rather than word, stimuli were used; until, however, matched lists of sentences suitable for children are available, for both visual and auditory reception, the word stimuli can serve our two purposes.

comprehension of spoken language

Once we have assessed the child's preferred channel, or channels, for receiving spoken language, then we must attempt to estimate his comprehension of this material. Our use of these results goes beyond its necessity for planning a remediation program for a child; the results are discussed with the child's teacher to help her understand the child's behavior and limitations in a classroom. We continue to emphasize our collaboration with the classroom teacher because of its crucial importance for a child; a child does not function in isolation and neither should we. A fragmented and disintegrated remedial program is wasteful and inefficient.

Peabody Picture Vocabulary Test (PPVT) The PPVT, a test of single word receptive vocabulary (Dunn 1965) was developed and used with normally hearing children as a measure of intelligence. For this population, it has been found to correlate highly with the scores obtained from other intelligence tests. However, since a primary effect of a hearing impairment is on language development, the PPVT cannot be employed as an IQ test with hard of hearing children. We use the test with such children to gain a quantitative estimate of their receptive vocabulary. We emphasize this point because of our concern that the Peabody scores obtained with hard of hearing children may be interpreted in intellectual rather than language terms.

Prior to administering the test, it is necessary to verify that the child's auditory reception has been maximized, by troubleshooting the hearing aid and by administering the test in a face to face fashion in a quiet room. The stimulus word is ordinarily presented orally in the carrier phrase, "Show me _____." The child is then required to select the one picture on the plate that best represents the stimulus word. If the stimulus is presented more than once, as may be necessary for some children, or if the child is asked to orally repeat the word to ensure that it has been heard correctly, these modifications from standard testing practices must be noted on the test form.

When using tests designed for normally hearing children on the hearing impaired population, we simply cannot be purists about our procedures if we hope to gain any useful information at all. One problem with the PPVT is that the tokens are presented in isolation, which excludes the normal possibilities of comprehending a word through situational and other linguistic cues. This format particularly affects the understanding of verbs, which are rarely heard out of context. This feature of the test is evidently no problem with normally hearing children, but hard of hearing children are masters at developing alternative strategies for comprehending words from contextual clues and depend much more upon such context for comprehension of unknown words. (This strategy can only take them so far and is the reason why they sometimes seem to make such "silly" mistakes in responding to oral messages.)

The receptive vocabulary score on the PPVT compares the hard of hearing child's age equivalent performance to a normally hearing child of the same chronological age. Thus a ten year old hard of hearing child who attains a 7 year 8 months score on the PPVT shows a gap of 2 years 4 months compared to the average normally hearing child. In conjunction with the normal standard deviation this score tells whether the result obtained is within normal limits (no more than two standard deviations) for a child of that specific chronological age. Beyond these numbers, however, the test can yield information on the kind of specific error patterns made by the child, such as with nouns (shoe, dog, bus), with verbs (sewing, submerge, descent), with categorizations (weapon, transportation, appliance), and with occupation titles (chemist, chef, sentry). The astute examiner—observing and questioning the child regarding errors—can discern his strategy for dealing with unfamiliar material, such as depending upon the process of elimination (if the answer is definitely not this or that picture then it must be one of the other two) and the use of associative clues (pointing to the picture of "store" by associating the unknown stimulus "mercantile" with a known word "merchant").

When explaining results to the classroom teacher, it is possible to relate the child's test performance to the difficulties he has, or will have, in comprehending orally presented classroom material. Subjects such as science and social studies may be especially difficult because of the rapidity with which new vocabulary is presented. This vocabulary deficit may be the reason for apparent behavioral problems in the classroom, such as not paying attention or disrupting nearby activities, simply because the child is being bombarded with words which are not understood.

For example, consider the following question, given on a 6th-grade drug test to an 11-year-old hard of hearing girl:

> A tiny amount of pure LSD can produce a sensation causing serious personality changes in the person who takes it. (T) or (F)

We have underlined the words which we predict that the child would have difficulty understanding, on the basis of her PPVT scores and our long personal involvement with her. She knows the concept being tested with this question, but simply does not understand the question itself. If there were just one or two new or difficult words in the question, she could perhaps comprehend its intent by the total context and answer appropriately. While up to this point she has been able to compensate for her vocabulary deficiencies and make acceptable academic progress, it is doubtful if this can continue unless the vocabulary limitations illustrated by this example are explicitly recognized and remediated.

Test of Auditory Comprehension of Language (TACL) This test (Carrow 1973) assesses the child's comprehension of the morphological and syntactic rules of spoken English. The word, phrase, or sentence is presented orally, and the child responds by pointing to the picture which best represents the stimulus. As with all other tests which require oral presentation, the examiner must often modify standard presentation practice so as to increase the likelihood that the child's responses reflect his current language status and are not simply errors in speech perception. The test may be administered with the examiner presenting the morphological markers at a normal rate and intensity—as with a normally hearing child—or by increasing, that is exaggerating, the intensity at which the markers are presented. The decision to administer the test with one or both methods should be made prior to the testing session, and so noted on the test form.

The interpretation of the results varies according to the mode of presentation, whether "normal" or "exaggerated." If the test is administered at a normal rate and intensity, the results illustrate the child's performance under ordinary conditions. In these situations, it may be the case that the child cannot hear unstressed morphological markers (/t/ or /z/, for example), and thus is responding on the basis of an insufficient acoustic stimulus. It is not possible to generalize with any assurance to the child's actual knowledge of these markers when this situation prevails. The results suggest the child's functional ability to comprehend the markers in a normal conversational situation (which of course provides many other linguistic and contextual cues for the comprehension of the grammatical information transmitted by the marker). Under these conditions, we cannot determine if the incorrect responses reflect the child's lack of knowledge of the grammatical marker, or simply if the salient acoustic information was not perceived.

When the marker is presented in an exaggerated form (increased intensity)—thereby increasing the likelihood that the child at least detects its presence—the results reflect the child's linguistic performance under more optimal conditions. A high score emphasizes the need to ensure that the child is receiving maximum high frequency information through his amplification systems. A low score indicates the need for language remediation activities in addition to amplification changes.

One cannot assume, however, that the child's knowledge of the grammatical rules of English can be completely defined by the TACL. Not only does the test not sample all the grammatical markers in the English language, but it should be recalled that the ceiling of the test is 6 years 11 months. For any child scoring at this relatively low ceiling, it is not possible to ascertain if he possesses the more sophisticated syntactical knowledge necessary to comprehend complex verbal material presented in a normal classroom. When such a child reaches the test ceiling, all that can be concluded is that he exhibits *at least* this age level facility with morphology and syntax.

The results of the TACL have implications for the hard of hearing child's classroom performance. The teacher's awareness of this inability to understand specific syntactical and morphological forms may positively influence the understanding of the child's social behavior (when he responds inappropriately because he did not completely understand the message), the expectations for academic performance (when the child's language ability is far below the level contained in his text books), and the presentation of oral material (when the child appears to be inattentive or fidgety). It may be that the child's failure to complete homework assignments, for example, may be caused by his poor comprehension of the language used to explain the work. We have often observed teachers presenting assignments, both orally and in writing, in language which exceeded the child's functional language ability. This is particularly noticeable when the assignment itself requires a language level which the child can manage, but where the directions are given in more complex language. The teacher may find by reducing the complexity of instructions, and asking the child to rephrase them for verification that these steps may improve homework and classroom performance.

The following example illustrates how directions can be simplified to ensure comprehension by the child. A normally hearing child was asked to read these directions from a workbook page to the entire class during a 7th-grade remedial reading class.

> Read the incomplete sentences at the left below. Then read the lettered phrases at the right. In each blank write the letter of the phrase that correctly completes that sentence. All the phrases will not be used.

The teacher (a very astute and sensitive one) then undertook to translate the directions in simpler language:

> You have a sentence here (points) that has no ending. In the right column (points) you pick the best ending for this sentence. Two of them you will not use.

Because concrete elements—such as pointing—were added, and simplified syntax used, the hard of hearing child was able to complete the workbook page, which was well within his functional language capabilities.

Durrell Paragraph Listening Test This test (Durrell et al. 1970) is not one which is ordinarily included in a speech and language assessment battery. We suggest its use for the purpose of simulating the linguistic demands made upon the hearing-impaired child during a classroom lesson, or during an extended conversation in which unfamiliar content material is being presented. The test consists of eight orally presented paragraphs of increasing difficulty, to which the child must respond by answering questions based on the content.

The test is most effectively presented in a setting which closely resembles a classroom situation. Thus, in an ideal setting, the test would be given to an entire class in which one or more hard of hearing child is also enrolled. The examiner should stand in approximately the same position the teacher assumes when giving instruction to the class, with the child also remaining in his accustomed position. The child's amplification system should be that routinely used in the classroom, whether personal hearing aids, or an FM auditory trainer. Unfortunately, this ideal situation is rarely possible because of the need to involve an entire class of normally hearing children. In most instances, the test is actually administered in a one to one fashion in a quiet room. The paragraphs and question should be read clearly and carefully, without special emphasis on the content words which may aid in answering the questions.

Because the test has no formal cutoff built into it, it is necessary to administer all eight paragraphs regardless of the child's performance. This takes approximately 35 minutes. The child responds to orally presented questions by filling in the bubble under the correct answer; random, guessing responses are scored and thus may give an inflated estimate of the child's actual status.

Regardless of the method of presentation (whole class or one-to-one), the test norms can be applied to estimate how the hard of hearing child compares to his normally hearing peers on this comprehension task. The whole class method has much more face validity, in that it closely replicates a normal classroom situation and permits a direct comparison with the child's hearing classmates. As indicated above, however, enlisting the child's entire class for this purpose is not always very realistic. However, valuable prognostic information can also be gleaned from results of the one to one presentation.

Poor scores in general on the test support the child's need for an intensive preview and review paradigm, in which the child is familiarized with the general content of a lesson and its specific vocabulary prior to the classroom presentation, and then given an opportunity to review the lesson subsequently. The behavior exhibited by the child when the test paragraphs become increasingly difficult can often assist the teacher in understanding the genesis of such problems as classroom inattentiveness, disruptiveness, and the "borrowing" of answers from the child in the next seat.

Consider the following verbatim paragraph which was presented by a 10th-grade teacher who was giving directions to his class (in which a hard of hearing child was enrolled) about the cancellation of a quiz and the scheduling of a test:

> We definitely will not have the quiz Monday. That's for sure. I want to finish what we're doing here today and I want to start the narrative. O.K. Reading that along with the oral questions based on the narrative. And we have one more listening exercise to do—comprehension in the workbook. After we finish this and we have the test, I'll review the chapter. Remember the bargain I made with you. Right. This test can count as two tests so I want to make sure that you are prepared for it. If not, some of you are going to bite the dust this semester.

Ten different information units are contained in this nine-sentence paragraph. It is easy to see how these syntactically complex instructions could cause confusion for a child who has reduced language skills, even to the extent that he might miss essential information.

It is also possible to adapt the Test of Auditory Comprehension (TAC), subtests 8 and 10, to serve the same purpose as described above for the Durrell—that is, to assess the child's comprehension in a format which resembles a classroom lecture or an extended conversation. Five paragraphs which were designed using vocabulary and syntax applicable for children in the primary grades, are available for oral presentation (seven if the two practice paragraphs are used). Instead of being graded in difficulty, they are equated for vocabulary and syntactical complexity so no paragraph is any more difficult than another. There are five orally presented questions for each paragraph with the response being the selection of one of four pictures. As the mode of presentation of these subtests differs from original use, the norms cannot be applied. Instead the percentage of correct answers can be interpreted as an indicator of the child's reception and understanding of connected speech when vocabulary and syntax are held constant.

production of spoken language

Our recommended analysis of spoken language includes the traditional areas of vocabulary, morphology, and syntax. We should like to extend our analysis of the child's language production, however, beyond these traditional categories and evaluate how effectively the child is able to use language for purposes of communication. Such information is very useful for teachers to have regarding hard of hearing children in their classes; they can thereby form realistic expectations regarding a child's ability to ask questions, formulate answers to the questions of others, and in general participate in class discussions.

A hard of hearing child needs facility in spoken language to interact socially with his peers. He just cannot get by using only single word expressions if he wants to be a participating member of a group. He must know how to take turns in a conversational exchange and how to properly adapt his language to reflect listener status. Unfortunately, while we would like to subject the use of spoken language to a standardized, sophisticated analysis, the assessment tools we have available only permit a cursory glance at this complex dimension of linguistic development. So we shall have to make do with what we have (keeping in mind that such non-standardized assessments as the Kretschmer and Kretschmer one referred to earlier are available and should be employed).

Developmental Sentence Analysis This test (Lee 1974) is used to assess the syntactic complexity of the child's spontaneous spoken language. Its analysis requires the elicitation of a comprehensive sample of the child's spontaneous output. More than any other test reviewed up to this point, the specific sampling procedure used and the rapport developed between the examiner and the child can greatly modify the obtained results. In order to elicit an adequate spontaneous language sample we have used such techniques as the following with some success.

(1) Try not to use pictures. If they are used, select those that allow the following kinds of questions: "What happened before this action occurred?", "What are the people saying to each other?", and "How do you think _____ is feeling?".

(2) Role playing can permit a conversational format without falling into a traditional question and answer routine. For example, we can ask the child to make believe he is a policeman giving a ticket, or a waitress in a restaurant, or a mother who is angry at her child for tracking in mud.

The point is not the specific technique used, but the need to evoke a representative language sample from the child. The quality of the analysis is totally dependent upon the adequacy of the sample. If a good one is not obtained, there is no point in proceeding any further with the analysis.

The transcription of the child's tape recorded language sample can be improved by repeating ambiguous utterances immediately after the child says them. It is easier to understand a child in person (through speech-reading, gestures, context, etc.) than a recorded version of the same speech. For example, when the third person singular is marked by /s/, but is weak or indistinct, the examiner may say "That's right, he walks up the stairs." Another possibility is for the examiner to take notes of such occurrences for later use.

Minor modifications in scoring the DSS language sample makes it possible to obtain additional pertinent information regarding the hard of hearing child's expressive language skills which can be used for planning remediation. The error mark (-) is used to indicate that a verb has been attempted and was incorrect. This results in a much higher score for the child who successfully uses simple present and past tenses than for the child who also has the ability to use the less complex forms, but chooses to express himself in a more sophisticated manner and, in doing so, makes more errors. Many hard of hearing children have been observed to attempt complex primary and secondary verb forms, such as "could have been," "have been going," and "started to fish," but in doing so, they may have eliminated part of the auxiliary verb or a critical verb ending. The fact that they attempt these complex forms is not acknowledged on the standard score sheet. By putting the complexity number of the attempted form over the error marker (7), it is possible to indicate at what complexity level errors occurred.

We also suggest that examiners consider adding an adaptation to the sentence score formulation given in the DSS manual. According to Lee (1974), if any aspect of the sentence is semantically or syntactically incorrect, a sentence point is not given. A hard of hearing child, however, is likely to make more than one such error per sentence; these additional errors are not reflected in the elimination of the single sentence point. Also, many of the errors are on forms that are not assessed by the DSS procedure (possessives, adverbs, and prepositions), so these errors are not considered in the scoring protocol in any other way but through the sentence point. If a child makes more than one error per sentence, or if the error relates to a form not included in the scoring procedure, it is useful for the examiner to include this information in their personal records. Our purpose in administering a DSS is not simply to derive quantitative measurements, but to help plan a remediation program. For this reason, it is helpful to indicate why the sentence point has been eliminated (for semantic errors, syntactic errors, or both). The tape recording of the child's utterances should be kept; this permits a longitudinal quantitative and qualitative analysis of the child's speech and language output.

The DSS overall score provides minimal information regarding the syntactic complexity of language used by hard of hearing children. More information is gained by analyzing the level of complexity of language that exists within each category. For example, it may be observed that a child produces all of his compound sentences by joining two simple sentences together with the conjunction "and" rather than using the more complex and more advanced linguistic structures of relativization, complementation, and embedding, or he may fail to substitute the appropriate pronoun for common elements (in a coordinate, compound sentence).

The DSS also gives the hard of hearing child credit for using forms that may be the basis of his linguistic deficiencies. For example, and in contrast to the example given above, many hard of hearing children substitute personal and indefinite pronouns for specific lexical items when they do not know the right word to use. Thus, they may use the words "that" or "this" or designate an item simply as "it" when a specific word is not in their vocabulary. In the DSS procedure, every instance of pronoun usage is scored, which results in an inflated complexity score. What this does is reward the child for a strategy he uses to circumvent his vocabulary deficits. The examiner must note these occurrences when interpreting the individual category performance of the child.

Other Measures of Language We have tried several other techniques for assessing spoken language in an attempt to circumvent problems inherent in using spontaneous language samples. The (1974) Carrow Elicited Language Inventory (CELI), which requires a child to repeat 51 sentences of increasing complexity, was employed in an attempt to assess language forms that were not spontaneously appearing in language samples elicited for the purpose of a DSS procedure or for a non-standardized language assessment. The test is based on the theory that a child will process the model sentence to be imitated through his own syntactic system.

Thus, modifications that appear in the child's version of the model presumably reflect the child's knowledge of the language principles which are being tested. If, however, the sentence to be imitated exceeds the child's verbal memory capacity, the rephrasings, reductions, or omissions which occur may be due to memory problems rather than syntactic limitations.

Another dimension is added to the test when it is used with hard of hearing children, since the child must also process the sentences through his deficient auditory system. Thus the cause of the resulting faulty imitative behavior becomes unclear (memory, linguistic, or auditory limitations). In addition, the test does not provide an opportunity to assess the child's knowledge of discourse rules (such as the need to provide a referent for a pronoun in a previous sentence) or the obligatory usage of certain syntactic forms (using present progressive verb to answer the question "What's happening?") since no spontaneous sample is obtained.

An additional technique, the Story Completion Test (Goodglass 1972) was also included on a trial basis in the test battery we administer to hard of hearing children. This test is designed to reflect the child's knowledge of discourse rules as well as the obligatory use of certain syntactic forms—the two factors cited above that are not assessed by the CELI. A short one- or two-sentence story is presented to the child with the last sentence left incomplete. The child completes the sentence based on the information he has received. A picture is used to help solidify the story line. The incomplete stories require the child to use a variety of morphological and syntactical forms in order to express the correct meaning. For example, one test item goes as follows: "I saw a purple car next to mine. I wanted to know who it belonged to. So I asked the policeman_____". A pilot study completed at the University of Connecticut (McNamara 1980) showed no significant difference in the child's use of specific syntactic forms through this test, imitation tasks (the CELI), and elicitation of spontaneous samples (DSS).

In another project completed at the University of Connecticut, the Story Completion Test was expanded to include the developmental hierarchy of syntactic structures used in Lee's Developmental Sentence Analysis. Forty-four revised items and pictures were devised and administered to hearing-impaired children in the public school. Our results showed that the procedure facilitated the assessment of the production of syntactic forms in an appropriate linguistic context. The revised test avoids many of the problems inherent in elicited imitation and analysis of spontaneous language tasks, such as memory restraints and inadequate language sampling.

As we previously stated, this battery that has been described includes those readily available tests that assess those communication skills necessary to function in mainstream classroom. New tests are constantly emerging from related disciplines which seem appropriate for use with hard of hearing children. As more mainstreamed children reach adolescence and are expected to grasp sophisticated concepts, the need has arisen to find tools that assess these higher level language skills. Three new tests seem to have potential use with this age group: Test of Adolescent Language (TOAL), the Clinical Evaluation Of Language Function (CELF) and the Fullerton Test of Adolescent Language. They need to be subjected to the same scrutiny given tests in the established battery in terms of presentation, adaptation, and interpretation before their general use can be recommended.

Several subtests of the Wechsler Intelligence Scale for Children (Weschler 1974) are useful tools for evaluating and quantifying several expressive and receptive verbal dimensions (as with the PPVT, we do *not* consider the resulting scores in relation to IQ, but to a level of language achievement). The vocabulary subtest assesses the child's ability to define words. The information subtest requires the child to answer specific questions on material he is assumed to have been exposed to and to have learned in school. The comprehension subtest assesses the child's ability to understand questions which require inferential reasoning to answer. The scaled score for each subtest permit the hard of hearing child to be compared with his normally hearing peers.

The Detroit Test of Learning Aptitude (Baker and Leland 1967) includes several subtests which we have used and found useful for the older hard of hearing child because this test includes norms for children up to age 18. The verbal absurdities subtest assesses the child's ability to recognize absurd verbal information contained in short spoken paragraphs. In the verbal opposites subtest, the child must provide the precise antonym to single word stimuli. The final subtest we have employed from the Detroit Test is the likenesses and differences subtest. Two stimulus words are presented orally, with the child having to tell how the words are alike and different.

Subjective Language Assessment Finally, we need some estimate of how effectively a child is able to use and understand language in its social context—that is his ability to employ the correct forms to establish contact with other people, to influence other's actions, to secure desired objects or experiences, and to obtain information. Learning to use language requires a sensitivity to the demands of the social context and the people in it (such as how and when to take turns speaking). This does not come naturally unless one has had a sufficient amount of linguistic exposure in different situations. Hard of hearing children have to be able to interpret the differences between "Is that door open?", "Don't you ever shut the door?", "The door is open." "Why don't you ever close the doors?", and "Shut the door!" when spoken by a parent or a teacher in different circumstances.

We take this ability to understand both the language forms and the intention of a speaker in particular situations (direct, indirect, on inferred commands) for granted in normally hearing children. The hard of hearing child, on the other hand, is likely to understand or be able to use only one or two linguistic forms in responding to the communicative intentions of others or to express his own intentions. He often may understand the words used by a person, but not the implied meaning.

Hard of hearing children frequently do not know the latest slang expressions, or understand jokes, riddles, or verbal analogies all of which act as a barrier to their effective use of language, particularly with their peers in a social context. We do not have standardized ways of judging a child's problems in the way he uses language in social situations. The clinician can gain an insight into them by observing the child in naturalistic situations and by devising experiences or using expressions to which the child must respond. Using a nonstandardized assessment of language behavior, the skilled speech/language pathologist can evaluate the child's status in a large number of pragmatic, semantic, and syntactic behaviors for which standardized measures are not available (Leonard, et al. 1978).

What should be obvious from this brief exposition into the language assessment of the hard of hearing child is its current makeshift status. Valuable information concerning a child's status can be obtained, but it is best not to depend too heavily on the results of any single test and to supplement formal test results with subjective impressions and nonstandardized analyses of language abilities.

assessment of speech production

Many of the tests traditionally used by speech-language pathologists to assess speech production skills can be used to measure these same competencies in the hard of hearing child. These include tests such as the Deep Test of Articulation (McDonald 1964), the Templin-Darley Test of Articulation (Templin and Darley 1969), the Goldman/Fristoe Test (Goldman and Fristoe 1969), and the Fisher-Logemann Test of Articulation Competence (Fisher and Logemann 1971). When used with hard of hearing children, one must ensure that it is the children's expressive status which is being evaluated, and not their ability or inability to understand what is required of them (naming pictures when the word is not in their lexicon, for example). These traditional tests have the advantage of being readily available in most public school systems. There is no reason why they cannot, with the qualification already expressed, be used for hard of hearing children.

The most comprehensive assessment procedure for evaluating speech production skills of hearing-impaired children was developed by Ling (1976; 1978) specifically for these kinds of children. Although it was primarily designed for children with severe and profound hearing losses, the test is also perfectly applicable for children with lesser degrees of hearing loss. The evaluation consists of examining the oral-peripheral structures and function, a phonological analysis (using the stimuli recorded during the DSS or other test of linguistic function), and a phonetic level evaluation. This latter stage involves the analysis of whether particular sound patterns are present, and whether they occur in different positions, in various vowel and consonant contexts, at different rates of utterance, and in changing combinations of alterations with other sound patterns. The difference between the phonologic and phonetic analyses may suggest phonological limitations in certain sound environments, or problems with the phonetic or phonologic transfer (carry over).

Since its introduction in 1976, the test has been widely used by teachers and clinicians working in special education settings for hearing-impaired children. It has not to our knowledge been used extensively with hard of hearing children in mainstream settings, although for many reasons it should be. In addition to presenting the evaluation procedures (and an impressive preliminary scholarly overview of the physiology of speech production and perception) Ling also discusses specific remediation steps associated with the findings of the evaluation.

Beyond this detailed analysis of a hard of hearing child's articulation deficiencies, there is still a need to gain some overall estimate of the intelligibility of the child's speech. It is perfectly possible for a child with even a severe articulation deficit to have intelligible speech, or for children with superficially similar speech evaluation results to manifest quite disparate degrees of speech intelligibility. This is an important dimension of the overall assessment of a hard of hearing child. He may have a lot to say, but if his peers and teachers cannot understand him, he will not have the opportunity to talk or be discouraged from talking. Such children will often avoid classroom discussions, or responses to a teacher's questions.

We have used the nine-point rating scale developed at the National Technical Institute for the Deaf (Subtelny 1975), but have found it does not have sufficient definition in the intelligible speech range to satisfactorily delineate speech production deficiencies of mainstreamed hard of hearing children. Another technique, first used by Hudgins at the Clarke School for the Deaf many years ago, is to have the hearing-impaired children read a list of words. Their speech intelligibility score would be the percentage of the words that normally hearing listeners can understand (or the reverse of the usual procedure in a speech discrimination test, where it is the listener and not the speaker who is being evaluated). The method is not used very much now, if at all, but it is one which still merits consideration. It is simple to administer and permits a very convenient way of conveying information about a child's speech intelligibility. It also offers a comparison between children and the same child's scores over time (for example, a score of 62% one year and a score of 76% the following year). The major problem with this testing procedure is that the words are spoken in isolation, and thus the influence of sentence context cannot be examined.

In a dissertation completed at the University of Connecticut, Seewald (1981) developed a test of speech production intelligibility which uses a sentence/multiple choice format. The child is recorded while reading a list of twenty-five sentences, with each one constructed so that a specific word in the sentence could be one of five possible words. The listener has the sentence frame in front of him with a blank indicating the key word. His task is to select the word the child actually uses in the sentence. The child's speech intelligibility score is the percentage of words correctly identified by the listeners. The list of sentences and the multiple choice word foils can be found in Appendix C.

Seewald also employed the speech production intelligibility rating scale developed at the National Technical Institute for the Deaf and correlated the results obtained by both methods for the eighty-four normally hearing and hearing-impaired children who served as subjects in his study. The correlation between the two procedures was extremely high (0.97), indicating that both methods of evaluating speech intelligibility reflected the same underlying attribute.

Regardless of whether one or all of these suggested methods for assessing the speech production skills in hard of hearing children are used, it is important to keep a yearly tape recorded log of the child's actual spontaneous speech. In the long run, it is this ability to transmit a message accurately that is the ultimate goal of any speech training program and it provides the only really significant comparison over time.

comprehension of written material

It is desirable to gain some insight into the child's comprehension and use of written language; some, but not all, of this information can be obtained from various academic achievement sub-tests. The Test of Syntactic Abilities (TSA) developed by Quigley and his associates (Steinkamp and Quigley 1976) specifically for hearing-impaired children provides the most comprehensive evaluation of their ability to comprehend linguistic structures in written form. The language dimensions evaluated include negation, conjunction, determiners, question formation, verb processes, pronominalization, relativization, complementation, and nominalization. It includes most of the structures that occur frequently in English and are important for reading comprehension.

The screening test was constructed to assess a student's general knowledge of syntactic structures and to identify any deficiencies in working with the various syntactic structures. There are twenty individual tests in the diagnostic battery with each test covering a single syntactic structure. The results of this evaluation can help the teacher understand sources of many of the child's reading problems and plan appropriate remedial programs.

○ ACADEMIC ACHIEVEMENT ASSESSMENT

A significant component of every hard of hearing child's Individual Educational Plan (IEP) is the results of academic achievement tests. The child is in school to be educated, and the results of such tests provide us with an estimate of how well we have succeeded in this purpose. School systems vary in the frequency that academic achievement tests are administered, the specific ones selected, and the personnel designated to actually administer the tests.

We suggest that the hard of hearing child be scheduled for achievement testing on a yearly basis even though the school system may not be required to do it this frequently for normally hearing children. For the hard of hearing child the need for continual reassessment of his class placement and monitoring of his education status is much more important than for a normally hearing child. There are those opponents of tests who deny that the child's test results accurately sample his actual knowledge, and that it only provides a measure of the test content itself. And there is merit to this argument. We do not consider such tests as infallible indicators of the child's academic status; certainly, the results by themselves should not be used to make critical educational decisions. Nevertheless, they are the best objective indices we currently have regarding a child's educational status, so for us to simply dismiss them entirely because of their imperfections does not demonstrate a helpful attitude. Through careful administration of achievement tests on a yearly basis, we can plot the child's academic progress, in relation to his previous scores and to his relative standing with normally hearing peers.

Most academic achievement tests are ordinarily administered to an entire class at one time. Group administration makes it difficult to ensure that hard of hearing children can hear and understand the directions. Whenever possible, these children should be tested individually, or in small groups, to minimize any complications arising from difficulties hearing and understanding the examiner.

We suggest that the achievement tests selected be the same ones usually administered to the normally hearing children in the school. The grade equivalency and percentile ranking scores obtained by the hearing-impaired children can then be directly compared to the scores achieved by normally hearing children. An additional score shows the child's relationship to his actual classmates on each of the subtests. If for any reason the conditions for administering a standard achievement test are altered (such as the time limits), they should be noted and the results interpreted accordingly.

The level of mainstreaming in the child's program as well as the child's communicative proficiency are deciding factors in selecting either a test normed on a normally hearing or on a hearing-impaired population. If the standard test is not deemed appropriate, then it is possible to use the Stanford Achievement Test which has been specifically adapted for use with the hearing impaired population (SAT-HI). Each of the language based subtests (vocabulary, reading comprehension, etc.) are presented one level below the usual level selected for presentation. Thus, it is possible to obtain a percentile score comparing the hearing-impaired child to other hearing-impaired children of the same age as well as a grade equivalent based on normally hearing children.

Interpretation of the test results is complicated by the fact that a number of achievement tests assign the same descriptive label to a subtest which requires widely different responses from a child or may actually be tapping different underlying skills. As an example of this occurrence consider four commonly used achievement tests: the California Achievement Test (CAT), the Iowa Test of Basic Skills (ITBS), the Metropolitan Achievement Test (MAT), and the Stanford Achievement Test (SAT). Each of them purport to measure vocabulary, spelling and language usage. In the vocabulary subtest, three of these require a child to read a stimulus word and select from four choices the word which has the same meaning. In the fourth test (SAT), the teacher dictates the word—which would present additional difficulties for the hard of hearing child.

In measuring spelling skills, the CAT requires the child to select one of four responses which best fits a blank space in a written sentence; the ITBS requires a child to identify one of four words as the correct spelling of one read by the teacher; the MAT requires spelling of a dictated word; and in the SAT, the child must identify a misspelled word from a set of four. Clearly, the label "spelling" is not tapping the same underlying skill for these four tests.

In language usage, the CAT requires the child to select one of four response possibilities which best fits a blank in a sentence; in the ITBS, the child must choose which one of three sentences is grammatically correct; in the MAT no individual language usage test is employed, but rather an overall category called "language" which combines usage, and knowledge of punctuation and capitalization—the former is usually harder for hard of hearing children than the latter two; and in the SAT, language usage is included in language arts, and requires the child to display knowledge of the relationships between different parts of a sentence.

It becomes the speech-language pathologist's responsibility to initiate a discussion of the child's test performance that takes into account the subtest format and presentation with the classroom teachers. The test results may reflect the child's hearing loss (difficulty in simply getting the message) or his underlying language deficiencies. In general, we would expect the hearing-impaired child to perform well on the analytic, concrete subtests such as math computation and spelling and poorly on those subtests which are language based (vocabulary, math word problems, reading comprehension). The evaluation process is not complete until these interrelationships and their implications for the child's day to day school behavior and performance is transmitted to the teachers. We emphasize a point we have already made and will be continuing to make: Test results should be used to develop or modify a child's educational plan and must impact upon school performance.

Some time prior to the scheduled date of the test, we advise that the speech-language pathologist review the vocabulary of the test directions with the child. This is not a trivial step; it is quite possible that a child's performance may be negatively affected because the written (or oral) directions are too involved for him to understand the tasks required. For some children it may be desirable to give them practice on the tests by using a similar or alternate form. As our purpose in administering these tests is to assess the child's knowledge of academic content, and not to assess whether he understands the means (the directions) by which this is accomplished, such a preview will increase the likelihood that the test results do indeed help satisfy our purpose. To empathize with the difficulties hard of hearing children can have with following test directions, we suggest that readers consider their own experiences in completing their own income tax forms or the innumerable other forms required in our increasingly bureaucratized society.

○ PSYCHOLOGICAL TESTING

Many of the same concerns we voiced regarding academic achievement testing also apply to psychological testing. It is common for schools to administer group intelligence tests at regular intervals throughout a child's school career. These tests can unduly penalize the hard of hearing child when they combine both the verbal and performance item to obtain a single IQ score without ensuring that the child has fully understood the directions. We suggest that hard of hearing children be tested individually by a qualified psychologist (in this context, qualified means one who understands the potential impact of a hearing loss upon performance). In order to rationally plan a child's educational program, some estimate of his intelligence is required. It is sometimes too easy to ascribe a hard of hearing child's poor performance to his hearing loss, when in truth, he may be functioning to the limits of his intellectual ability.

In selecting IQ tests appropriate for the hard of hearing child, it is necessary to use those that permit separation of the verbal and performance portions, each of which can then be broken down into a number of subtests. Reporting just a full-scale IQ, that is the average of the verbal and performance items, penalizes the hard of hearing child. No one should accept such a score as representing the child's intellectual status. The scores on the verbal portion of an IQ test should not be reported as the "verbal IQ"; it can be reported as a verbal score, but such a score should not convey any connotation of intelligence.

The scores the child achieves on the performance section of an IQ test gives us our best estimate of the child's intelligence. However, inadequate attention to verbal variables can still affect the validity of this component.

The directions given to the hard of hearing child must be understood by him; it is not enough for an examiner to mumble the directions while reading them from the test booklet. The child must understand the task required of him, whether he can do it or not, if the test is to have any validity. For such a child, we suggest that the examiner supplement verbal directions with demonstration and gesture to ensure that the child understands what is required of him.

The Wechsler Intelligence Scale for Children (WISC-R)—which is separated into verbal and performance portions, each with a number of subtests in each area—has been used extensively with hearing-impaired children. Other tests have been developed specifically for children with hearing problems, such as the Arthur Adaptation of the Leiter International Performance Scale (AALIPS) and the Nebraska Test of Learning Aptitude (NTLA). This latter test provides norms for deaf children when the instructions are pantomimed, and norms for normally hearing children when verbal directions are used. A comprehensive review and analysis of appropriate psychological tests and their necessary adaptations when they are administered to the hearing-impaired can be found in Boyle (1977). In general it is best to administer a battery of tests which delineate the child's potential and learning style rather than rely on a single test.

During the psychological tests, it is important that the examiner be alert to the possible presence of other problems in addition to the hearing loss. It is tempting, but somewhat simplistic, to routinely ascribe a hard of hearing child's poor achievements to the presence of a hearing loss. The child may also be slightly retarded, or exhibit specific perceptual or language disabilities. The majority of hard of hearing children do not exhibit multiple problems—and, in our judgment, many who do are showing the sequelae of inappropriate and/or delayed management—nevertheless these instances do occur and must be considered. When a child is multiply handicapped, it is very difficult to separate out the influence of the individual components; each component must be dealt with on its own terms while trying to minimize the compounding effect of the other factors (for example, ensuring that auditory factors are under control when working with a child who also manifests a learning disability).

○ CLASSROOM OBSERVATIONS

This dimension of a child's performance is often overlooked when conducting a comprehensive evaluation. In many ways, however, this is the pay-off, the culmination of all our efforts with a child. It is simply not possible to judge whether a hard of hearing child's educational placement and performance is appropriate—and whether or not additional measures should be taken—unless we observe him, his teachers, and his peers, in a natural setting. It may take several observations during different activities to truly get the feel for this child as a participating member of the classroom. For example, to watch him only during seat work would not provide a sufficiently diverse sample of his total adjustment. If we coupled this observation, however, with his behavior during a reading group and a general class discussion, as well as in gym, math, social studies, we can more realistically ascertain whether or not this child's special needs are being met and whether the comprehensive performance assessment accurately reflects the child's performance in a natural situation.

In approaching any teacher regarding the schedule for a classroom observation, speech-language pathologists (assuming that this person will be the most frequent observer) must stress that the focus of their attention is the hard of hearing child and how best to help him in the classroom. They must emphasize that their job is to support the teacher in efforts to educate the child in a regular classroom, not to supplant the teacher's primary role vis à vis the child. These observers must express their willingness to continue to make specialized expertise available to the teacher on an ongoing basis throughout the school year because all are part of the same team whose responsibilities pertain to the education of the hard of hearing child. Teachers in no way should be made to feel as if their competency is being assessed or questioned. In a properly run school district, the teacher should have already received some orientation regarding the special problems posed by a mainstreamed hard of hearing child before the child is enrolled in the classroom. This orientation, the acquiescence of the principal, and a sensitive session with the speech-language pathologist (perhaps over a cup of coffee in the faculty lounge) should be sufficient to elicit a willing acceptance of the speech-language pathologist's classroom visits by the teacher.

The following outline enumerates those observations which help to further describe the hard of hearing child as he performs in a classroom environment. Later, in the section on classroom management we shall discuss them more fully.

(1) The participation of the child in classroom activities and in classroom discussions
    a. Does he ever raise his hand in response to a teacher's question?
    b. Does he raise his hand simply in imitation of the other children but not really know the answer to the question posed?
    c. Does he volunteer for any classroom activity?
    d. Is he able to follow the speaker in a classroom discussion, or is he out of it?
    e. Is he reticent about speaking because of his awareness of his speech difficulty?

(2) The interactions between the child and his teacher
    a. Does the teacher avoid verbal interactions with the child (perhaps because of his difficulty)?

b. Does the teacher ignore the child as long as he behaves (even though he needs help)?
c. Are the teacher's expectations regarding communicative and academic performance less than they should be?
d. Is the teacher visibly impatient with the child's problems?
e. Does the teacher make any efforts to help the child gain acceptance from his peers (perhaps with a unit on hearing loss)?

(3) The adaptation of the teacher's classroom style

a. Does the teacher modify verbalizations appropriately (simplifying language, repeating, and paraphrasing when necessary)?
b. Does the teacher modify when it is not necessary (or underestimate the child's ability to comprehend complex language)?
c. Does the teacher repeat the answers of the other children?
d. Does the teacher use a sufficient number of visual-aids (blackboard, pictures, demonstrations)?
e. Does the teacher verify the child's comprehension of instructions?
f. Does the teacher encourage the child to ask on the spot questions?

(4) The interactions between the child and his classmates

a. Is he a social isolate or does he have friends?
b. How do his friends communicate with him (normal language, simplified, gestures, or some combination)?
c. How does the child handle situations in which he does not understand what is being said?
d. Does anyone make an effort to ensure that the child can follow the general content of a social conversation?

(5) The child's strategies for learning and processing content material

a. Does he take notes or does he concentrate on listening?
b. Does he use note takers if he cannot do both simultaneously?
c. Does he ask questions when he does not understand?
d. Is he able to formulate specific and appropriate questions?
e. Does he require written information to supplement verbal material?

(6) The use of an FM auditory trainer by the teacher and child

a. Should an FM system be recommended (see auditory management)?
b. Is the teacher using it appropriately?
c. Does the child inform the teacher when it is not being used correctly (such as transmitting to child when unnecessary)?
d. Does the child inform the teacher when something is wrong with the unit?

(7) The source, level, and location of speech and noise sources relative to the child

a. What is the overall SPL noise reading at the child's location, with normal ongoing classroom activities?
b. Is the teacher's speech received by the child at a positive signal to noise ratio (estimate, when child is using a hearing aid or FM receiver as a hearing aid)?
c. Is the child sitting next to a noise source?
d. What are the major noise sources?
e. Can they be eliminated (except for the children)?

It is apparent that this outline cannot cover every eventuality of classroom behavior that is pertinent for the education of the hard of hearing child. Sensitive clinicians will observe many variations on these themes. The task is to integrate the results of formal tests with the child's observed classroom behavior and communicates their combined implications to the team required to plan a child's educational program. The formal test results, by themselves, are a little sterile; supported by on-site observations in the classroom, however, we are able to imbue our comprehensive performance evaluation with meaning whose relevancy can be much more acceptable to teachers than scores on tests. We do not consider any comprehensive performance evaluation of a hard of hearing child complete unless classroom observations are included as an integral, and vital, component.

○ PARENTAL INTERVIEW

Under Public Law 94–142, parents are required to explicitly agree, by affixing their signature, to the individual educational plan developed for their child. We can preclude possible difficulties in their acceptance of the IEP—show them that we are their allies and not their adversaries in the effort to improve their child's lot—by bringing them into the management process from the very beginning as a contributing factor in the comprehensive performance evaluation.

In the past, there has been a tendency to simply inform them of the therapeutic program being offered to their child without sufficient consideration of their input into the process. By enlisting their involvement at this early stage, by informing them of the objective test results and our subjective impressions, we can gain a great deal of insight into their aspirations for their child. Their goals for their child, their perspectives regarding his difficulties, can serve the dual purpose of helping us refine the details of the IEP and ensure their informed cooperation in its fulfillment. It is difficult for professionals to appreciate how intimidating the atmosphere of a formal IEP team meeting can be for parents, where they see the future of their child decided by people who do not have the same emotional investment in the child as they do. A prior parental interview, as the initial contact in an ongoing series of interview/counselling/information sessions can help assauge their fears.

In initial contacts with the parents, we suggest a listening rather than a questioning strategy. We can, by asking the parents to "tell us about _____, what do you think about how he is doing?" not only elicit most of the information we need from them for IEP purposes, but also convey our real concern and interest in their child (which should hopefully continue during the entire management process). Within this general approach, one can still pose specific questions to clarify certain details. At the conclusion of the interview, we should be able to gain some insight into the following considerations:

(1) What are the parents' judgments regarding the child's academic performance to date? Do they feel the need for additional assistance, with an explicit focus on the child's special needs?

(2) What are their attitudes towards the child's hearing loss? Do they understand its behavioral implications, or do they think that the child is sometimes "putting them on"? Are they still working through their feelings about having a handicapped child and finding it difficult to take positive actions?

(3) Is the responsibility regarding their child's welfare shared by both parents, or does the burden fall on just one? Do the parents have congruent or conflicting views and expectations regarding the child's behavior and future?

(4) What are the parents' vocational/academic goals for the child? Do they see him going on to college, or to a trade school? (We are definitely not suggesting the superiority of one over the other.) Is he going to work on the family farm, or in the family business?

(5) Does the child have a regular circle of friends? A best friend? What is his position in the group (a fully participating member, just tolerated, or a "pet")? How do they view the child's social status?

(6) Do the parents consider their child to be a happy child? What do they see as his strengths? Does he have any hobbies, or particular interests? Does he seem to have a positive or a negative self-image?

We have, as should be evident from the above considerations, a rather broad perspective on what information is appropriate in a comprehensive performance evaluation. We do not, however, see how it is possible to formulate a relevant IEP without this information. We simply cannot erect a barrier between school and home considerations and expect that either will proceed satisfactorily.

○ THE INDIVIDUALIZED EDUCATION PROGRAM (IEP)

Every professional in the United States who works with handicapped children knows of the Education for all Handicapped Children Act, better known as Public Law 94–142. This law has revolutionized the education of all handicapped children by requiring, as it does, the completion of an individualized educational program (IEP) for each child. Every school system in the United States has an IEP form which must be completed on each identified handicapped child. Although the details may vary, all the forms are required by the law to report specific assessment and management considerations.

Up to now our presentation of these considerations have of necessity been somewhat general since they could not be directed at a specific hard of hearing child; at the time an IEP is completed, however, these general considerations have to be translated into a concrete program for each such child. In this presentation, we will not attempt to cover all the details and ramifications of an IEP as it is outlined in P.L. 94–142 and interpreted by the National Office of Education and various state agencies (Dublinske 1978; Dublinske and Healey 1978). We shall, rather, review the components of an IEP from our personal perspective, adding those qualifications, comments, and iconoclastic reservations which appear justified on the basis of personal experiences.

case coordinator

For every handicapped child, somebody has to assume the responsibility for developing and implementing an IEP. For the hard of hearing child in the regular schools, we suggest that this person be either the speech-language pathologist, the teacher of the hearing-impaired, or the educational audiologist. We can make a case for all of these individuals, but when all three are available in the same school system, we prefer the educational audiologist. This person should understand the nature and total implications of a hearing loss more than any other professional in the school system. Furthermore, a well-trained educational audiologist should have enough background in the operations of the rest of the educational team (the speech-language pathologist, the regular and special teachers, and the school psychologist) to enable him to serve as an information conduit and synthesizer. In distinction to the speech-language pathologist and the teacher of the hearing-impaired, most of whose time is rigidly scheduled in tutorial therapy blocs throughout the school day, the educational audiologist's school day is usually more flexible. Built into the educational audiologist's schedule is time for classroom visitations, consultations, and tests of uncertain duration; ordinarily he develops his own schedule and thus can make time to assume the case coordinator role.

We prefer, incidentally, to use the term "case coordinator" rather than the frequently used term "case manager" in order to suggest that this role does not imply any superiority vis à vis other IEP team members; in any event, an IEP team should include an administrator, perhaps the director of special education or his designate, whose responsibilities *do* include overall supervision of the case.

If the school system does not employ at least one educational audiologist (which in our judgement, it should if the child is to receive the "appropriate" education mandated by Public Law 94–142), then the speech-language pathologist is the next most suitable person in the school system to serve as case coordinator for a hard of hearing child. We do not mean to automatically exclude teachers of the hearing impaired from assuming this role. Our reasoning, as we indicated earlier, is that the focus of their training concerns the deaf, not the hard of hearing child. We make a distinction between these two types of children, and thus, the personnel who must serve them. We are, however, less concerned with the title any professional or individual carries, and more concerned with the competencies they possess—their ability to do the job. Our primary responsibility is the hearing-impaired child, not the promotion of any professional group.

The case coordinator must be familiar with the provisions of Public Law 94–142—as implemented in the school system—and the mechanics of completing an IEP. The coordinator must, with the concurrence of their supervisor, schedule the team meetings and arrange for the attendance of all required and desirable personnel, ensure that all necessary assessments are completed prior to the meeting, and take continuing responsibility for the implementation of the team's recommendations. This latter step is particularly important; nothing of any real significance for a child happens just because we write it down on an IEP form.

The value of having educational audiologists serve as the case coordinator is that he is in continuing contact with a child, his teacher and all other support personnel and thus in a position to judge whether the team's recommendations are being carried out. Not the least among his responsibilities is sensitizing the school personnel to a hard of hearing child's hidden problems. It is easy to underestimate the problems experienced by these children by observing their superficially normal behavior or believing that the provision of hearing aids will solve their problems; or perhaps go to the other extreme, and categorize them with "deaf" children and insist that the children require a more restrictive educational placement. Herein lies one of the main values of standardized tests for the hard of hearing child, not only to suggest areas for therapeutic intervention, but to objectively demonstrate the impact of the hearing loss upon the child.

Prior to the IEP meeting, the case coordinator should review the process of the IEP development with the parents. They must be apprised of their rights under the law and realize that the law permits and advises them to serve as equal partners in developing an IEP for their child. If they desire to bring a private consultant to the meeting, a lawyer, or a member of a parent advocacy group, they must be permitted to do so. The case coordinator must demonstrate to the parents that the team is truly interested in the welfare of their child and try to preclude an adversary stance between the parents and the professionals. The parents must be informed of the procedural safeguards built into the law which protects their rights. They have the right to inspect and review all the educational records of their child related to the proceedings of the IEP team; they can obtain, at no cost to them, an independent evaluation if they disagree with the one conducted by the local school authorities; they can request that the State Educational Agency convene a formal hearing on the IEP team's recommendation; they can, if they are still not satisfied, institute civil court proceedings. If the case coordinator fulfills his role sensitively and professionally and if all the staff in the school in contact with a child develop a relationship of mutual trust and confidence with the parents, few families will feel the need to take advantage of the foregoing procedural safeguards.

IEP content

Every IEP must include statements regarding the child's present level of all aspects of performance. These statements (based on the results of the comprehensive performance evaluation discussed earlier) must describe the child's level of accomplishments in as specific, objective, and quantitative a manner as possible. Vague and generalized statements regarding the child's accomplishments are not acceptable. The results of all standardized tests should be reported in age or grade equivalent scores, percentiles, raw or standard scores; any way, in other words, in which the child's performance can be objectively related to the test norms and to his own accomplishments at an earlier or later time. Standardized tests, however, only sample some of the dimensions of communicative performance; they do not completely define the child's overall communicative performance; they do not completely define the child's overall communicative capacity. In an IEP, the description of a child's performance should not be limited to statements arrived at only from the results of standardized tests.

The nonstandardized assessment of language behavior has received a respectable review by a number of authorities in the field of speech-language pathology, education of the deaf, and psycho-linguistics (Bloom and Lahey 1978; Kretschmer and Kretschmer 1978; Leonard et al. 1978). Such assessments are viewed as essential mechanisms for understanding a child's linguistic system so that personalized intervention strategies can be devised. The particular area in which a child has problems can be defined—such as his inability to comprehend indirect requests or the proper use of articles —and sufficient relevant tasks devised to achieve a numerical baseline estimate of his current status. It is not possible, however, to quantify every dimension of a hard of hearing child's educational, communicative, and psycho-social performance (nor, in our judgment, may this even be a desirable objective, considering the ethical implications in attempting to perfectly classify, and therefore categorize, human beings).

In attempting to conform to the requirement that this statement of a child's performance be described in a quantitative form, there is the possibility that clinicians will limit assessment to dimension that can be so described and exclude those that, while more relevant, cannot easily be defined in a quantitative form. (Perhaps this is done to satisfy some local and state authorities whose supervisory emphasis too often seems to focus on the form rather than the content of an IEP.) The clinician who admits to an inability to quantitatively define the child's status in some dimension, but proceeds to describe it as clearly as possible, is serving the child better and meeting the clear intent of Public Law 94–142 much more than the one who ignores or overlooks the problem area.

All IEPs require a statement of specific short-term and annual goals, written in a manner so that a reader will know what is to be done, who is to do it, when it will be completed, and the criteria and evaluation method to test whether the goal(s) have been accomplished. Additionally, any special services required by the child to further the goal of "appropriate" education for him, must be included (such as tutoring, classroom amplification, special tutoring, and follow-up audiological and otological evaluations). If the child requires a change in his educational placement (into a more or less restrictive setting), then this recommendation must be fully justified in the IEP.

The heart of the IEP team's deliberations for a child is contained in the above considerations. They must be made on the basis of the child's needs and not whether they are immediately available in the school system or whether budgetary restrictions prohibit the implementation of certain recommendations. First, the child's needs are defined; then reality has to be confronted in an attempt to carry them out. The best opportunity for obtaining the services required by a hard of hearing child is when the IEP is formulated. This is the time that all the involved professionals as well as the parents present their case for the child's management based on assessment of his performance.

Just about every such child will require speech and language intervention; the frequency and intervention method used must be described. Visits by the speech-language pathologist and the educational audiologist to the child's classroom and consultation with his teachers must be scheduled. Most such children will require academic tutoring; the frequency and material employed in this tutoring must be designated and coordinated with the teachers and the speech-language pathologist. A specific tutor, or the method of acquiring one, has to be designated. All audiological management considerations have to be spelled out and included in the IEP. The projected date for the initiation and termination of any recommended service must be stipulated; if interim assessments and objectives are considered desirable, their dates too should be included in the IEP. If possible, nothing should be left to chance or open.

A very common annual goal for a hard of hearing child is to increase his vocabulary. Such a goal, in IEP terms, can be written as follows:

Annual Goal	Instructional Materials	Goal Evaluation
To teach the child to comprehend 300 new words with 100% accuracy	Teacher-made material, crossword puzzles; social studies, science, and reading textbooks; classroom handouts	Pre- and postcriterion referenced vocabulary tests

A very common short-term goal for a hard of hearing child is to attempt to increase their perception of the phoneme /s/. Such a goal, in IEP terms, can be written as follows:

Short-term Objective	Instructional Materials	Evaluation of Short-term Objectivation
To use residual hearing for the perception of /s/ with 80% accuracy	Hearing aid which responds to frequencies above 4000 Hz (as demonstrated by aided audiogram); Pre-recorded audio tapes; language master; teacher-made materials	Pre- and posttests using high frequency word lists and nonsense syllables

In Table 3–3, we provide a check list of possible services required by hard of hearing children for use by the case coordinator and the IEP team. The check list is not designed to supplant or in any way modify the IEP form. We suggest that it be used as a guide to ensure that the appropriate services pertinent to the management of a hard of hearing child (based on our work and experiences) are considered when planning a program for a particular child.

A number of the items—such as the comprehensive speech and language evaluation, academic achievement tests, psychological evaluations—must be completed on every child prior to the IEP team deliberations. During the IEP meeting, all the items which are required for a particular child should be checked; another check should be placed in the "present" column for those services the child is currently receiving, or had already received. The details of any required (or recommended) service should be transferred to the IEP form. For example, if partial or follow-up audiological or speech and language evaluations are thought necessary during the course of the school year, the nature and schedule of the specific tests are to be detailed on the IEP form. Or if tutoring or some specific therapy is required, the who, what, when, evaluation, and criterion requirements referred to earlier must be completed.

The reader will note twenty eight items in the check list. There are also two blank items, since we cannot claim that we have had experience with every possible relevant service for a hard of hearing child which could be appropriately included in an IEP. This is a large number of potential services, which may possibly be pertinent to hard of hearing children. *All* should at least be considered for *every* hard of hearing child (and for some of the items, his parents).

We must confess to a slightly jaundiced view of the requirement to specify the annual goals and the short-term instructional objectives in strictly behavioral terms. Some of the objectives we have seen written on IEP's remind us more of the occult than a humanistic therapy endeavor. We have never

TABLE 3-3

A Program Development Check List

The list is designed as a guide to ensure that the appropriate services pertinent to a particular child are at least considered when developing an IEP.

	REQUIRED	PRESENT
1. Comprehensive speech and language evaluation		
2. Partial/follow-up speech and language evaluation		
3. Comprehensive audiological evaluation		
4. Partial/follow-up audiological evaluation		
5. Academic achievement tests		
6. Psychological evaluations (including an individually administered performance scale)		
7. Classroom observation		
8. Personal hearing aid(s)		
a. Individualized electroacoustic adjustments		
b. Daily troubleshooting		
9. FM Auditory training system		
a. Individualized electroacoustic adjustments		
b. Daily troubleshooting		
10. Otological examination/treatment		
11. Acoustical treatment of classes		
12. Vocabulary (classroom and environmental)		
13. Language therapy (syntax and morphology)		
14. Language therapy (inferential reasoning, problem solving, usage)		
15. Speech therapy (phonetic/phonological)		
16. Speech therapy (quality, prosody)		
17. Preview-review tutoring		
18. Notetaker		
19. Assigned "buddy"		
20. Staff orientation		
21. Peer orientation		

TABLE 3-3 Continued

	REQUIRED	PRESENT
22. Career counselling		
23. Psycho/social counselling		
24. Extracurricular social activities		
25. Parental contacts/counselling		
26. Parent group		
27. Alternative educational placement		
28. Other:		
29. Other:		

understood how it is possible to specify that a child *will* understand or employ some linguistic form or usage correctly after a certain period of therapy. Though such goals are not legally binding, their endorsement by the panel of "experts" constituting the IEP team can easily raise expectations in the parents and in the child, which a later qualification—saying that some percentage of a given goal has been met—will do little to ameliorate consequent disappointment. We prefer a little more humility (or perhaps honesty) by the professionals when goals are set. Perhaps we should use the word "try" rather than "will" (which is really what we are doing, anyway). It is one thing to set attainable therapeutic objectives and work toward fulfilling them, it is quite something else to shroud these objectives with an aura of scientific objectivity and thereby obscure the many unknowns associated with any human interaction.

placement alternatives

The hard of hearing children to whom this book is primarily devoted are those in their regular classes but still receiving supplemental special services and instruction. For some hard of hearing children, this may not be sufficient. Their communication and educational problems may be too severe, the resulting social isolation may be too acute for them to receive an "appropriate" education in a mainstream educational setting. One of the most difficult decisions an IEP team has to face is the question of a placement alternative for such a child. These decisions have to be faced, however, and not simply postponed year by year. If the assessment shows that the child cannot sufficiently comprehend the classroom lessons, if he is unable to communicate effectively with the teacher and his peers, if the educational achievement and language gap with his peers is getting larger, if he is a social isolate or perhaps adopted as a "pet" by well-meaning peers, the IEP team must consider a placement alternative for the child. We are obligated —professionally and ethically—to confront this decision; we cannot permit the tragedy of a child unhappily and inappropriately placed in a regular class to continue. Better alternatives must be found or created.

Unfortunately neither the IEP team nor any of its members has the power to make programmatic changes in a school system. Nor is there any effective way of instituting such changes for just one child. Creation of effective placement alternatives requires a view from on top, either from the local education agency, an intermediate (regional) educational agency, or from the state department of education, depending on the population of hearing-impaired children who require a similar placement alternative within a given system. Such alternatives include: a special resource room for hearing-impaired children who, however, spend most of their time in a regular class; a special class with the children spending some time in regular classes (the above can be combined in actual practice); self-contained classes in regular school; to self-contained classes in a public day school; a private day school; or residential schools. In our experience, while "the view from on high" may be favorable for such alternatives, a great deal of prodding from below is frequently necessary to bring them about. The first two alternatives are particularly applicable for the kind of child we are considering in this book, though we have—and correctly so in our estimation—recommended more restrictive placements for some hard of hearing children.

In order to make such a decision, the exact number of children who require a particular alternative must be determined; a room or rooms must be found in a central school location; the staff and the children in the school must receive an orientation program; a qualified teacher(s) must be found to staff the resource or self-contained special class; supplemental assistance must be on site or on call (the speech-language pathologist and the educational audiologist); travel arrangements must be made; and, parental meetings must be scheduled for all those who will have a child in this particular alternative. In other words, when the IEP team makes a recommendation for a placement alternative to the parents, they should have some assurance that it is presently, or shortly will be, available. One cannot inform parents that their child is not properly placed in a school and not be able to offer a suitable alternative. The factual basis for the team's decision should be conveyed to the parents, but not as a *fait accompli.*

It may be necessary to schedule several meetings with the parents, bringing in other teachers who have had experience with the child, as well as the prospective teacher of the resource room or special class, and corroborative assessments may have to be scheduled before the parents feel comfortable or accepting of the recommendation. The point must be made that this does not represent a failure for the child. Different children have different needs, and their child's needs require a more intensive or in some way different program. We do not want to lay a load of guilt on the parents or make them feel that they or their child has failed. Often, parents are relieved when they realize that there is a viable educational alternative available for their child. Most are very well aware of the educational, communicative, and social problems of their child; the placement alternative offers them some hope that the situation can improve in the future.

A parent's group is a crucial component of the placement alternative. A hard of hearing child in a regular class may not know any other hard of hearing children in his age range; his parents, also, will not ordinarily have any sustained contact with parents of hard of hearing children. A group for parents of mainstreamed hard of hearing children, is, therefore, difficult to organize and continue. Not having any program "umbrella" in common, they go their own isolated way and do not have the support of others who have problems similar to theirs.

When, however, a child is placed in a resource or special class, the "umbrella" is available to help form a parent group. Such a group offers more than an opportunity for the professionals to convey information to the parents. It allows the parents, probably for the first time, the chance to express, exchange, and deal with the unresolved feelings of having a handicapped child (Luterman 1979). Unless the speech-language pathologist and/or the educational audiologist are competent to lead such a group—and currently not many are—it is necessary to collaborate with our colleagues in psychology and social work in its management. In our judgment, the recommendation for more restrictive educational placement should include an explicit statement regarding the formation and staffing of a parents' group.

case reports

As we have stressed on several occasions, the dissemination of our results to the proper school personnel is an integral component of the evaluation. This dissemination may be both in an oral and written form. In our ongoing contacts with the teachers and school administrators it is necessary that we translate and expand the findings and implications of the performance evaluation; moreover, since the evaluation is itself a continuing process, we must keep our colleagues apprised of continuing developments.

Several examples follow with the major emphasis on interpreting test results for the classroom teacher. Table 3–4 presents the comparative results for two children of similar chronological age on a battery of speech, language, academic, and psychological tests. The reduced performance of child #1 relative to child #2 is clearly evident.

In Table 3–5 we show the information we would communicate to children's teachers based on these results. The first column indicates the areas of major deficiencies; the second column predicts the type of classroom behavior which can be expected; and the third column makes concrete and

TABLE 3–4

A Comparison of Two Children (C.A. 11–1), with Equivalent
Hearing Losses, on the Speech/Language Evaluation, Achievement
Testing, and Psycho-Social Assessment (Grade 6 Placement)

Comments: Child #1 has consistently lower scores than Child #2, especially on language loaded tasks. Both children score at grade level or at age level on analytic concrete tasks (math). Both children demonstrate a reduction in the comprehension of spoken language, with Child #1 showing the greater delay. Child #2 makes better use of residual hearing, which results in an improvement in reception of speech in a combined mode. The effect of the language deficiency is apparent on the achievement testing and the psychological assessment.

TEST NAME	CHILD #1	CHILD #2
PPVT	7–1	9–8
TACL	6–11*	6–11*
Durrell	7–0	10–4
PBK		
Look	52%	56%
Listen	56%	74%
Look and listen	72%	88%
DTLA		
Likenesses and differences	6–4	14–3
Verbal absurdities	5–4	11–8
DSA	errors on simple verbs	uses complex verbs
Speech intelligibility	78%	87%
TSA (only below 75% recorded)		
Relativization	68%	all above
Complementation	54%	cut off
SAT (grade equivalent)		
Vocabulary	3.1	4.9
Reading comprehension	4.0	6.1
Word study skills	6.7	10.4
Math concepts	5.9	11.1
Math computation	7.4	9.7
Math applications	3.0	5.8
Spelling	7.1	8.4
Language	4.9	6.0
Social science	3.7	5.8
Science	4.1	5.4
WISC–R (10 ± 3 normal range)		
Verbal		
Information	5	7
Comprehension	4	8
Similarities	7	7
Arithmetic	3	5
Vocabulary	4	4
Performance		
Picture completion	13	15
Picture arrangement	14	14
Block design	12	10
Object assembly	8	11
Coding	9	10

*ceiling

TABLE 3-5
Information Conveyed to Teachers, Based on Results Given in Table 3-4

It is advisable to supplement this written outline with oral explanation

CHILD #1

Test Results	Classroom Behavior	Teacher Suggestions
1. Verbal comprehension is low PPVT TACL Durrell SAT [Vocab] [Read comp] [Math appl] [Social sci] [Science] WESC-R [Inf] [Comp]	Child will have difficulty with material presented in lecture-type format. Also will have trouble with the language-based subjects (reading, science, social studies, math word problems) that have heavy emphasis on new concepts and vocabulary.	1. Use visual demonstration of material. 2. Give child an outline of the presentation prior to the class. 3. Use visual display such as writing on board, using overhead projector. 4. Write key words on board. Also topic changes. 5. Give material to tutor a week prior to the presentation to preview vocabulary and concepts. 6. Check child's understanding through questioning. 7. Verbal presentation should be at normal rate and loudness, using a paraphrase version when necessary.
2. Reading comprehension is low TSA Relativization 68% Complementation 54% SAT [Vocab] [Read comp] [Math appl] [Social sci] [Science]	When the child is reading, he has difficulty understanding complex sentences, i.e., those that have clauses. He also has reduced vocabulary through the written mode. This is not surprising: the child has based his reading skills on his general depressed verbal language ability. Therefore, he will have trouble fully understanding written material, especially test questions, science and social studies textbooks.	1. Check child's comprehension of what he reads through question and answer format. 2. Have child answer content questions with his book shut so he cannot visually scan for the answer. 3. Keep instructions in simple syntax and ensure child has understood task. 4. Suggest tutor preview the content of assignments before the child attempts independent work.
3. Use of auditory skills is depressed PBK Listen 56% Look and listen 72%	Child needs multi-sensory classroom presentation in order to learn the academic material. He will have trouble following a class discussion involving a number of persons. When visual cues are eliminated, he receives only a portion of the message. Films, filmstrips, and tape recorded material will be difficult.	1. Face child when speaking: do not write on board and talk simultaneously. 2. Use visual aids. 3. Seat the child in a favorable place where the visual and auditory factors are optimal, taking into account the teacher's position. 4. Reduce room noise sources. 5. Consider use of FM system to reduce the interference of noise, distance, and reverberation. 6. Preview movies and filmstrip with tutor.

TABLE 3–5 Continued

	7. Direct classroom discussion by calling on the next speaker by name, and repeating the content of the message.

CHILD #2

Test Results	Classroom Behavior	Teacher Suggestions

1. Verbal comprehension is lower than expected for chronological age
  PPVT 9–6
  TACL ceiling
  Durrell 10–4
  Detroit
  Verbal Absurdities
  11–8
	Even though this child's academic skills are at or above grade level, his reduced vocabulary does effect his ability to understand verbal presentations with the facility or depth of his peers. He has difficulty with multiple meanings, idioms, and abstract ideas.	1. Have tutor preview and review vocabulary of academic subjects.
		2. Present speech/lang. pathologists with conversational vocabulary, needed to participate fully in classroom discussion.
		3. Optimize classroom listening situation to ensure child has opportunity to hear the rich verbal input.

specific suggestions to the teacher to assist them in working with the children. It is advisable to supplement the written outlines of Tables 3–4 and 3–5 with an oral explanation to the children's teachers to ensure that the information is understood and can be applied.

SUMMARY

In this chapter we have presented and discussed the elements of a comprehensive performance evaluation of a hard of hearing child. Beginning with the audiological definition of the child's hearing loss—the reason we are concerned with him in the first place—and ending with the parents, who are the most important figures in the child's life, we have stressed the need to evaluate his status as objectively as possible. Since many of the evaluation tools we utilize were not designed for children with hearing losses, we have pointed out that examiners must occasionally modify the standard instructions for administration and interpretation in an attempt to gain a more valid insight into the child's actual problems.

We have not presented a prescribed battery of tests. We are more concerned with the general dimensions which must be evaluated because our perspective concerns communication demands made upon hard of hearing children in a regular school. Tests are viewed as a preliminary step to management and not as ends unto themselves. Unless they can be clearly related to a management program, they are simply a wasteful burden to the children.

Finally, a theme that pervades this entire chapter is the absolute necessity to communicate implications of the comprehensive performance evaluation to all who are educationally involved with the children.

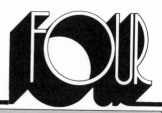

Remediation

○ AUDIOLOGICAL MANAGEMENT

Our first and indispensable objective in planning auditory management for hard of hearing children is to provide them with the maximum amount of salient speech acoustic information consistent with their hearing loss for as many hours during the day as possible. All other technical and organizational details and considerations follow from this objective. We do not mean to imply that other types of management considerations are irrelevant or unimportant, but that they must be based upon the full exploitation of a child's residual hearing and not serve as more or less ineffectual substitutes for our major goal.

It is not trivial or simplistic to point out that the hard of hearing children we are dealing with are handicapped precisely because they suffer from impaired hearing. This is the source of the communication and academic difficulties they display (reviewed in Chapter Two). By capitalizing on their residual hearing, we are, in a sense, heading some problems off at their source. In order to most effectively learn their lessons in the classrooms, they have to hear them; and the better they hear them, the more they are going to learn.

As we have already stated, these sentiments may appear to be simplistic, but we make no apologies. No factor, in our judgment, has been so sadly lacking from management practices for hearing-impaired children as the auditory factor, yet no program can hope to be truly successful unless it is founded on appropriate auditory management. In the following sections, we shall consider audiological management from the perspective of the simple model presented in Figure 4–1.

A number of interacting factors are seen to underly the final product of our efforts—maximizing the child's aided residual hearing. The first such factor is the speech signal itself; it is the sounds of speech that we want to deliver to the children and, therefore, the prospective teacher/clinician must be generally familiar with its acoustic and perceptual characteristics.

The language code conveyed by the acoustic signal is also, properly speaking, a component of an auditory management model. It is not included here because the major purpose of this section is elucidation of factors which must precede, and which set limits to, auditory linguistic development. The remediation of language, as a separate factor, will be covered in a later section of this book.

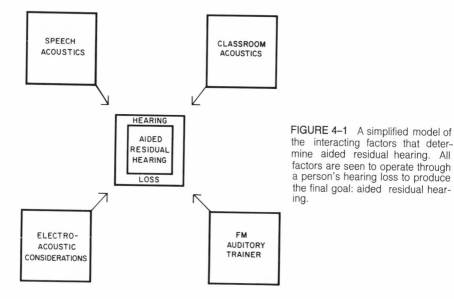

FIGURE 4-1 A simplified model of the interacting factors that determine aided residual hearing. All factors are seen to operate through a person's hearing loss to produce the final goal: aided residual hearing.

This speech signal is delivered to children in a classroom setting; the effects of the acoustic conditions existing in such settings upon a child's perception of the speech signal is the second factor which must be considered. We shall, therefore, be reviewing the concepts of noise and reverberation, their separate and interactive effects upon normally hearing and hearing-impaired children, and some simple steps which can be taken to reduce their impact upon speech perception.

Next, we must concern ourselves with the electroacoustic characteristics of amplification systems. The speech signal, as modified by the classroom acoustics, is transmitted through such systems before it is delivered to the ears of the children; so it is necessary to understand the potential contribution amplification systems make upon the child's ability to perceive speech sounds. In this section we shall include a brief description of the types of hearing aids available, acoustic changes which can be produced by earmold modifications, and troubleshooting considerations.

The interaction of these three factors upon the specific hearing loss exhibited by a child creates the final product—that is, the child's residual hearing. We emphasize that this product is simply the raw material of auditory perceptual development and that this material by itself does not guarantee that a child will make the most use of residual hearing. It is difficult to see, however, how any hard of hearing child can effectively employ his residual hearing for the development and utilization of communication skills unless he is supplied with the greatest possible degree of relevant acoustic information.

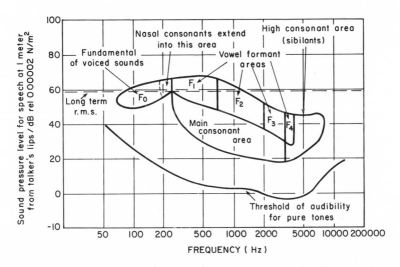

FIGURE 4–2 Spectral regions occupied by the major components of various speech sounds. (Richards 1973, reprinted with permission.)

Finally, we will conclude our presentation of auditory management with a discussion of wireless FM (frequency modulated) auditory training systems. We are specifying this type of system only because of a conviction that it is the only amplification system now available which can be used effectively by a hearing-impaired child in the public school system. Logically, this would be included in the Classroom Acoustics section since such a system was designed to overcome the negative effects of classroom listening; we include it here as a separate component to emphasize that the proper selection and use of an FM system can protect and ensure the maximum contribution of the three previous factors.

Our intention is not, particularly in regard to the topics of speech acoustics, classroom acoustics, and electroacoustics, to present comprehensive coverage. As already stated, we view this simple model as a mechanism for organizing a logical progression of auditory management factors into sufficient detail to communicate their relevance and interactions.

speech acoustics

The general spectrum of the speech signal can be seen in Figure 4–2. Before we discuss the major components of the spectrum, we should like to observe that it is plotted on an SPL scale (re 0.0002 microbar) rather than a hearing threshold level (HTL) scale (re "normal" hearing). To clinicians who are accustomed to viewing audiograms, plotting the speech spectrum in SPL terms may appear to be an unnecessary complication. In our

123

judgment, however, the ultimate convenience of being able to plot all the necessary dimensions of acoustic performance on the same reference level outweighs any short-term complications. For example, the electroacoustic performance of hearing aids and the acoustic conditions in classrooms are both ordinarily described in SPL terms and thus can be made congruent with speech acoustic measures. Moreover, given the increasing trend for selecting hearing aids in respect to their electroacoustic parameters (Ross and Tommassetti 1979), it will be useful for teachers/clinicians to become conversant with the SPL scale and its relationship to the familiar audiogram.

In Figure 4–2, the average binaural sound-field thresholds are represented in the lower curve. As can be noted, the frequency response of the normal ear is such that there is greater sensitivity between about 500 and 8000 Hz than at either extreme. A number of very important features of speech signals are apparent in the figure. The intensity of vowels is seen as generally greater than that of the consonants, and the intensity of the vowel formants is seen as decreasing as frequency increases. The main energy of both the voiced and voiceless sibilants extends to about 8000 Hz.

There is about a 30 dB spread between the weakest and the strongest speech elements at every frequency location; thus, communicating the intensity of a speech signal with a single figure, say 65 dB SPL, is misleading. In fact, the vowel peaks will extend about 12 dB above, and the weakest consonants, to 18 dB below, any such single figure used to represent the average intensity of a speech signal. This 30 dB range serves as a target sensation level to be provided hard of hearing children with the use of amplification.

The figure also shows the general decline in speech intensity as frequency increases. The average SPL at 3000 Hz is about 20 dB less than at 500 Hz. There is also a total 50 dB range between the strongest components at 500 Hz and the weakest components at 3000 Hz and higher. The possible problem this intensity decline could have on speech perception is partially overcome by the greater sensitivity of the normal ear at these higher frequencies.

Finally, the acoustic cue provided by nasal consonants (produced by resonance in the nasal cavity) can also be noted from the figure. Particularly for a child with a severe loss this energy can provide important cues for the perception of speech.

The average values of the fundamental frequencies and the frequency locations of the first three formants of 10 American English vowels for men, women, and children can be found in Table 4–1. Considering the results for the male speakers as the base, it can be noted that women's fundamental frequency averages approximately 85 to 90 Hz higher, while the children's are a full octave higher.

TABLE 4-1
Fundamental Frequencies and Formant-Characteristics of Ten American English Vowels

		i	ɪ	ɛ	æ	a	ɔ	U	u	ʌ	ɝ
FUNDAMENTAL FREQUENCIES (Hz)											
	Men	136	135	130	127	124	129	137	141	130	133
	Women	235	232	223	210	212	216	232	231	221	218
	Children	272	269	260	251	256	263	276	274	261	261
FORMANT FREQUENCIES (Hz)											
F_1	Men	270	390	530	660	730	570	440	300	640	490
	Women	310	430	610	860	850	590	470	370	760	500
	Children	370	530	690	1010	1030	680	560	430	850	560
F_2	Men	2290	1990	1840	1720	1090	840	1020	870	1190	1350
	Women	2790	2480	2330	2050	1220	920	1160	950	1400	1640
	Children	3200	2730	2610	2320	1370	1060	1410	1170	1590	1820
F_2	Men	3010	2550	2480	2410	2440	2410	2240	2240	2390	1690
	Women	3310	3070	2990	2850	2810	2710	2680	2670	2780	1960
	Children	3730	3600	3570	3320	3170	3180	3310	3260	3360	2160
FORMANT RATIOS											
F_3/F_1	Men	8.48	5.10	3.47	2.61	1.49	1.47	2.32	2.90	1.86	2.76
	Women	9.00	5.77	3.82	2.38	1.44	1.56	2.47	2.57	1.84	3.28
	Children	8.65	5.15	3.78	2.23	1.33	1.56	2.52	2.72	1.87	3.25
FORMANT AMPLITUDES (dB)											
L_1		−4	−3	−2	−1	−1	0	−1	−3	−1	−5
L_2		−24	−23	−17	−12	−5	−7	−12	−19	−10	−15
L_3		−28	−27	−24	−22	−28	−34	−34	−43	−27	−20

From H. Levitt 1978. "The Acoustics of Speech Production," in *Auditory Management of Hearing-Impaired Children*, p. 70. M. Ross and T. G. Giolas, eds. Baltimore: University Park Press. Reprinted by permission.

The vowel /i/ is composed of both the lowest first formant (270 Hz) and the highest second formant (2290 Hz). The fact that it is frequently confused with /u/ by many hearing-impaired children with high frequency hearing losses is explained on the basis of the similarities between their first formants—that is, because F1 of /i/ (270 Hz) and /u/ (300 Hz) are so close in frequency and because F2 of /i/ (2290 Hz) may not be audible to a hearing-impaired child, the two sounds may be heard as the same and therefore no discrimination can be made between the two vowels.

Not shown in the table is the bandwidth of the formants; it should not be supposed that formants are comprised of the single frequencies given here. On the average, the bandwidth of the first formant is approximately 50 Hz, with the bandwidth of the second and third formants slightly larger. Therefore a hearing-impaired child may be able to perceive part of a formant band and use that information for vowel identification and discrimination.

The correct perception of vowels by the normal listener is made based on the relative formant frequencies—that is, the formant relationships are such that the ratio of F1 to F2 of a specific vowel is relatively constant for all speakers, but it is different across vowels. For example, the ratios (F2/F1) of the vowel /i/ are as follows:

Men: $2290/270 = 8.48$
Women: $2790/310 = 9.00$
Children: $3200/370 = 8.64$

It can be seen that the ratios are relatively equal for each speaker group. Comparing the ratios between two vowels shows that they are quite different:

/I/ $1990/390 = 5.10$
/U/ $1020/440 = 2.32$

With this information, one can begin to appreciate that the perceptual task of a listener in attending to vowels and their adjacent consonants is to focus on the relative, rather than the absolute, values of a speech signal.

Table 4–2 gives the normal sensation levels of thirty-four English phonemes. The first column gives the average sensation level of each phoneme in respect to the threshold of hearing. The second column gives the level at which the phonemes can just be identified.

It will be noted that the consonant /θ/ can be recognized when its *average* level is below the threshold of audibility; this supports the point made earlier that representing a speech signal with a single intensity level can be misleading. In this instance, it is presumably the *peak* energy in the phoneme that cues the appropriate perception. The third column is the average of the two previous columns; this one shows that the range between the weakest phoneme in English, /θ/, and the strongest, /ɔ/, is about 25 dB. Our goal with frequency selective amplification is to make both of these phonemes audible to children.

The spectra of fricative consonants are given in Table 4–3. Note the high frequency composition of these phonemes, particularly the /s/. This phoneme has little energy below 3500 Hz. Until quite recently hearing aids rarely provided usable amplified sound beyond approximately 3000 Hz. Therefore this phoneme was inaudible to hearing-impaired children, even those who possessed significant amount of usable residual hearing in the frequency range of 3000 Hz and higher.

Ability to hear the /s/ has syntactic as well as phonemic implications. Some examples of morphological and syntactic information carried by the /s/ are: (1) the plural marker, for example "lamp" vs. "lamps"; (2) the possession marker, for example "Mark's marbles"; (3) the third person singular construction—for example, "She walks home"—and in differentiating the present from the past tense——for example, "She puts it away" vs. "She put it away"; (4) contractions—for example, "it is" vs. "it's," "let us" to "let's," and "what does" to "what's."

The first column shows relative levels as measured with respect to the threshold of audibility. The second column shows relative levels measured with respect to that level at which the sound is just recognizable. The third column shows the average of these two measures. All data are in decibels. Inasmuch as relative levels are shown, the least intense sound, $/\theta/$, was chosen as the reference and its average level was arbitrarily set to 1 dB.

RELATIVE SENSATION LEVEL (dB)	RELATIVE LEVEL RE: THRESHOLD OF RECOGNITION (dB)	AVERAGE (dB)	SPEECH SOUND	
26.0	26.0	26.0	ɔ	(sought)
25.6	26.0	25.8	ɑ	(calm)
25.5	26.0	25.8	aɪ	(sigh)
25.2	26.0	25.6	ɑʊ	(now)
25.6	24.9	25.3	oʊ	(soap)
23.4	26.3	24.9	a	(half)
25.2	23.2	24.2	æ	(sat)
23.1	24.1	23.6	u	(foot)
24.4	19.5	22.0	ɛ	(set)
19.3	24.2	21.8	eɪ	(day)
22.0	21.5	21.8	ɝ	(third)
21.9	20.3	21.1	u	(food)
18.6	21.5	20.1	ɪ	(sit)
19.5	18.6	19.1	l	(low)
15.4	22.3	18.9	i	(seat)
14.9	19.8	17.4	ŋ	(sing)
14.9	19.2	17.1	ʃ	(shed)
13.2	15.7	14.5	tʃ	(child)
12.8	12.7	12.8	n	(no)
9.7	15.7	12.7	dʒ	(jump)
11.4	11.1	11.3	m	(me)
10.1	12.4	11.3	t	(ten)
8.9	12.9	10.9	g	(gate)
9.8	11.3	10.6	k	(key)
10.2		10.2	ð	(then)
4.9	13.8	9.4	d	(den)
9.9	7.7	8.8	h	(home)
7.6	7.6	7.6	z	(zero)
4.8	9.7	7.3	b	(bend)
6.6	7.4	7.0	p	(pen)
7.4	6.1	6.8	v	(vine)
9.6	3.7	6.7	f	(fine)
8.4	4.1	6.3	s	(said)
4.7	−2.8	1.0	θ	(thin)

From H. Levitt 1978. "The Acoustics of Speech Production," in *Auditory Management of Hearing-Impaired Children*, p. 76. M. Ross and T. G. Giolas, eds. Baltimore: University Park Press. Reprinted by permission.

The acoustic composition of the other consonants is of a lower frequency than the fricatives. Since the majority of hard of hearing children possess better hearing at low frequencies than the high frequencies and since it is much easier to reproduce the lower frequencies with a hearing aid than the

TABLE 4–3

The Spectral Range and Shape of the Fricatives

The spectrum of the voiced cognates of these phonemes are similar, except for an additional voiced element superimposed on the fricative component and additional low-frequency energy in the vicinity of the fundamental.

PHONEME	SPECTRAL RANGE	SPECTRAL SHAPE
/f/	1500 to 7500	Rather flat over range
/s/	3500 to 8500	Little energy below 3500 Hz, peaks at around 4200, flat to 8500
/ʃ/	1600 to 7000	Little below 1500 Hz, peaks at 2200, 2800, and 4000
/θ/	1400 to 8000	Flat spectrum

higher ones, we can easily ensure detection of lower frequencies if we can ensure detection of the higher frequency consonants. The professional's knowledge of the acoustic characteristics of speech permits auditory training activities at a level and significance somewhat more relevant than requiring a child to differentiate between the sounds of bells and drums.

Table 4–4 provides another kind of overall view of the acoustics of speech (Gerber 1974). What this table shows is the relationship between different bands of speech and the percentage of speech power and speech intelligibility contained in those bands. These data were obtained on adults with normal language development, and not on congenitally hearing-impaired children who are endeavoring to learn language. Nevertheless, the relationships shown in the table, whose basic validity has been confirmed by many filter studies over the years, can enable us to appreciate the instrinsic capacity of the different bands of a speech signal to convey speech information.

Note that the low frequencies, under normal circumstances and for normal hearing adults, carry little of the intelligibility of speech but much of its

TABLE 4–4

Relationship Between the Percentage of Speech Power
and Speech Intelligibility Contained in Various Frequency Bands

FREQUENCY RANGE	SPEECH POWER %			INTELLIGIBILITY %		
62 to 125	5 ⎤			1 ⎤		
125 to 250	13 ▶	60		1 ▶	5	
250 to 500	42 ⎦		95	3 ⎦		
500 to 1000	35			35		
1000 to 2000	3 ⎤			35 ⎤		
2000 to 4000	1 ▶	5		13 ▶	60	95
4000 to 8000	1 ⎦			12 ⎦		

From S. Gerber 1974. *Introductory Hearing Science*, p. 244 Philadelphia: W. B. Saunders Co. Reprinted by permission.

power. These relationships support our focus on efforts to render audible to hard of hearing children as many of the high frequencies as their hearing losses permit.

In making this point, we do not mean to imply that the lower frequencies are useless. On the contrary, they help listeners recognize the emotional state of a speaker (anger, love, fear, embarrassment, etc.), (Ross et al 1973) assist in monitoring vocal output, help improve oral speech perception, and provide some important spectral cues to children whose residual hearing is limited to the lower frequencies. The value of the prosodic aspects of speech (intonation, stress, and duration), which can be conveyed by the low frequencies, also should not be underestimated. We emphasize the high frequencies simply because in the development of hearing aids, initially designed for use by adults, the high frequency acoustic needs of children still developing their language have not been given sufficient emphasis.

It is time to restate the caveat with which we began this section. We have here provided a simplistic and static view of a dynamic dimension. Speech is quintessentially the product of dynamic articulatory activities, with the majority of its acoustic/perceptual clues derived from phonetic assimilation and co-articulation. Thus, the static framework of speech acoustics that we have presented here omits the predictable acoustic modifications that occur in different phonetic environments and upon which normal speech perception is heavily dependent. Many of these dynamic cues for perception are also available to hearing-impaired listeners, and although their exposition is not feasible in this book (Pickett 1980) we would like to briefly note one that is of paramount importance and relevance to hard of hearing children.

Second formant transitions (and the third as well, but this is of less importance to hearing-impaired children) are direct reflections of the movement of the articulators to and from the consonant restrictions preceding and following each vowel. Each such movement in consonant articulation has a characteristic physiological effect upon the dynamic articulatory status of adjacent vowels. These articulatory movements modify the resonance characteristics of the entire vocal system in a unique fashion for each combination of adjacent vowel and consonant. These are seen acoustically as rapid frequency shifts to and from the steady state formant values given in Table 4–1.

Since speech is ordinarily syllabic, with consonants and vowels following one another in the normal flow of speech, these rapid frequency shifts—or formant transitions—are a normal component of the speech process. These transitions serve as powerful cues for perceiving the place of articulation of the consonants, particularly the stop consonants, which generally give hearing-impaired individuals a great deal of difficulty. The spectral energy (bursts of energy related to the release of the articulation) of these stop consonants are of a fairly high frequency (though not as high as /s/) and thus they are frequently inaudible, or audible in only a limited fashion, to a child with a high frequency hearing loss or one who wears a hearing aid with a limited high frequency range. These characteristic transitions of the second formants are of lower frequency than the burst energy of the plosives, and thus they can enable a hard of hearing child to correctly identify the presence of specific consonants which he cannot hear. That is, the child can detect the frequency shift in the vowel formant even though the high frequency energy associated with a particular consonant is not itself audible. Readers can verify this effect for themselves by uttering such nonsense syllables as /eep/, /eet/, and /eek/, and not exploding the final consonant but simply placing the articulators in the proper position. The /ee/ should sound different each time.

In brief, the reader should be aware that a speech signal incorporates multiple acoustic cues for the correct perception of speech sounds. Using any or all of them, however, is dependent upon speech being made audible; even the judgment of the lack of sound, such as when a child cannot detect a high frequency fricative, depends upon the perception of the audible acoustic frames of such phonemes. This consideration justifies our efforts to maximize the amplified sensation level of speech and rationalizes the usefulness of the view of speech acoustics presented here.

classroom acoustics

The speech signal produced by the teacher, or any other speaker, must travel a certain distance in the classroom before it reaches the hearing-impaired child. Therefore, the acoustic conditions existing in the classroom will have an effect upon the quality of speech signals received by the child. If the room is noisy and reverberant, much of the speech energy is going to be masked or otherwise distorted before it reaches the child; if he is some distance from the speaker, these effects will be greater than if he is close. In this section, we will discuss the classroom acoustics component of our auditory management model.

That classrooms are typically noisy places needs little elaboration here. Just how noisy they are, however, will often be surprising. The average sound pressure level found in several studies indicate that children have to learn in noise levels in excess of 60 dB SPL (Sanders 1965; Paul 1967). As part of the UConn Mainstream Project, we have measured the noise levels existing in forty-five classrooms in which a hard of hearing child was placed, and in sixty two speech-language rooms in which individual therapy/tutoring took place. The results are shown in Table 4–5.

The measures were taken during the normal school activities in the rooms and were measured on both the A and the linear scales of a sound level meter. The scales differ mainly in the additional weight given to the lower frequencies in the linear network. The A scale is closer to how the

TABLE 4–5
Average Noise Levels and Standard Deviations in 45 Classrooms and
62 Speech Rooms in Which Hard of Hearing Children were Placed

The measures were made under normal classroom conditions, with the other children
present.

LOCATION	NUMBER	"A" SCALE dB	S.D.	LINEAR SPL	S.D.
Classrooms	45	60	7	64	8
Speech rooms	62	49	9	55	10

normal ear actually hears the sound because the normal ear is also relatively insensitive to low frequencies (see Figure 4–2).

These results support the common observation regarding the poor acoustic conditions existing in classrooms. The mean results are bad enough; but when one considers the magnitude of the standard deviations, it is apparent that fully a third of the classrooms where, at least, sixty hard of hearing children were being educated (one to each classroom at a minimum) demonstrate SPLs in excess of 70 dB. These figures should be compared to the goal of achieving sound levels of about 35 dB on the A scale (in empty classrooms with normal activity in adjacent areas; our results were obtained with the children present).

Reverberation is another form of noise and can be even more detrimental to speech perception than noise produced by other sources. It is defined as the prolongation of sound after the source has ceased vibrating, and it is a function of the type of surfaces in a room. Hard concrete, ceramic tiles, wood walls, and ceiling reflect most of the sound energy, while porous surfaces (rugs, drapes, cork boards, acoustic tiles) absorb much more of the sound energy. The longer the reverberations continue, that is the longer the reverberation time, the greater its detrimental effect upon the perception of speech in classrooms. Reverberation time is defined as the length of time required for a specified sound to decrease 60 dB after the source has ceased.

A good figure to strive for is an average (125, 250, 500, 100, 2000, and 4000 Hz) reverberation time of 0.5 seconds. With durations longer than this, speech understanding begins to suffer considerably. What happens is that the strongest elements in the speech signal, that is the vowels, overlap in time and mask the later-arriving, weaker consonantal elements in speech.

As we have seen above, these high frequencies are particularly important for speech understanding and thus every effort should be made to reduce reverberation time. The actual reverberation times measured in classrooms are usually in excess of this recommended 0.5 seconds, reaching an average of 1.2 seconds in some studies (reviewed in Ross 1978).

The absolute levels of the noise and reverberation times are not so important as the signal to noise ratio (in this case the intensity of speech as

TABLE 4–6

Speech Discrimination Scores for Twelve Hard of Hearing
Children Under Noise and Reverberant Conditions

REVER-BERATION TIME (sec.)	SIGNAL-TO-NOISE RATIO (dB)	NORMAL HEARING	UNAIDED HARD OF HEARING	AIDED HARD OF HEARING
0.0	quiet	95	88	83
	+12	89	78	70
	+6	78	66	60
	0	60	42	39
0.4	quiet	93	79	74
	+12	83	69	60
	+6	71	55	52
	0	48	29	28
1.2	quiet	77	62	45
	+12	69	50	41
	+6	54	40	27
	0	30	15	11

From T. Finitzo-Hieber and T. W. Tillman 1978. "Room Acoustics Effects on Monosyllabic Word Discrimination Ability for Normal and Hearing-Impaired Children," *J. Speech Hear. Res.* 21, 440–458. Reprinted by permission.

compared to the intensity of the background classroom noise) in regards to effects on the perception of speech in a classroom. When the intensity level of the direct speech signal reaching a child or the microphone of his hearing aid (prior to its first reflections) is much greater than the totality of the noise and reflected sound at the same location, speech perception is enhanced. When it is not, the child will not be able to use his residual hearing effectively no matter how carefully the hearing aid(s) has been selected.

All studies which have investigated the actual signal to noise ratios existing in classrooms have consistently found the ratios to be typically unfavorable, ranging from plus 1 to 5 dB—that is, the speech is only 1 to 5 dB greater than the background noise level (Sanders 1965; Paul 1965; Ross et al. 1973).

While normally hearing children may be able to function adequately under such conditions (though this is an arguable proposition), hearing-impaired children cannot. The evidence clearly shows that hearing-impaired individuals are susceptible to greater absolute and relative effects upon speech discrimination than normal hearing people under the same conditions of noise and reverberation (Tillman, Carhart, and Olsen 1970; Gengel 1974; Finitzo-Hieber and Tillman 1978). This effect is apparent in Table 4–6 (data from Finitzo-Hieber and Tillman 1978).

Note from the table that in every condition of noise and reverberation, separately and in combination, the scores of the hard of hearing children are poorer, and become relatively worse, as the listening conditions deteriorate. For example, when there is no reverberation, the scores for the normally hearing drop 35% (from 95% to 60%) while the scores of the hard of hearing children drop 46% (from 88% to 42%). Under the poorest reverberation conditions (1.2 seconds, which is not at all unusual in classrooms today), the scores of the normally hearing children drop 47% (from 77% to 30%), while those for the unaided hard of hearing children also drop 47% (from 62% to 15%). With hearing aids, because of the imposition of reduced fidelity compared to the unaided condition (keeping in mind that the signal to noise levels were equalized in the aided and unaided conditions), the scores drop even more, to a horrendous low of 11%.

Every effort should be made to reduce the noise levels existing in classrooms in which hard of hearing children are enrolled. Noise levels of 64 dB SPL and reverberation times approximating 1.2 seconds are simply not acceptable. The most efficient procedure to reduce the noise levels and the reverberation time would be to sound-treat the entire classroom, for which it would be desirable to secure the services of a knowledgeable builder, or in difficult cases, an architectual acoustician.

Certain measures are obvious, however (Olsen 1977). Rugs on the floors and acoustic tiles on the walls and ceiling (preferably a dropped, low ceiling) will make an immediate, discernible difference in the classroom. Drapes over windows and the liberal use of cork boards can help when installation of acoustical tiles is not possible. We have seen creative teachers create interesting designs of colored egg cartons on the walls, with not only decorative, but favorable acoustical results.

The noise sources in the classroom should be identified, and steps should be taken to eliminate or reduce them (in spite of occasional temptation, we do not recommend eliminating the primary source of noise in classrooms —the children). Air conditioners and heating systems can be major sources of noise; it is possible to reduce the noise produced by these devices without impairing their operating efficiency. Overhead projectors, gaps under the hallway door, and windows opening on a busy thoroughfare are other common sources of noise in a room. The list can be extended almost indefinitely.

The first and most important step, however, in reducing excess noise levels and reverberation times in a classroom is to increase the sensitivity of classroom teachers and administrators to their terribly negative effect upon the speech perception abilities of hard of hearing youngsters.

Possibly the most powerful procedure which teachers/clinicians can use to assure maximal reception of speech by hard of hearing children in classrooms is to simply reduce the distance between their mouths and the microphone of the hearing aid. This phenomenon is graphically illustrated in Figure 4–3.

In accordance with our previous discussion, the figure assumes a 66 dB SPL speech level three feet from a talker, and 60 dB SPL of ambient noise equally distributed throughout the classroom. As can be noted, there are substantial increases in the signal to noise ratio as the distance between the talker and the microphone/child is reduced. At 4.5 inches from the

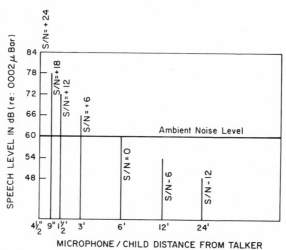

FIGURE 4-3 The effect of distance from the speech source on the signal-to-noise ratio. An ambient noise level of 60 dB is assumed to exist in the room.

speaker's lips (which is a good location for the microphone of an auditory trainer), the signal to noise ratio is a positive and acceptable 24 dB.

There is no magic about these results and the underlying concept; the essence of it is that the intensity of a speech signal increases as distance from the speaker decreases, while ambient noise tends to be fairly equally distributed throughout a room (except in the immediate location of noise sources). We will elaborate on this concept in the FM auditory training section of our auditory management model.

electroacoustic considerations

The next component in our auditory management model is electroacoustic considerations. We use the term "electroacoustic" rather than hearing aids and auditory trainers to emphasize that our main concern is with the performance characteristics of these devices and not with the manufacturer's name they bear. We are interested primarily in the quality of the amplified sound they are able to provide and only secondarily concerned with such other features as cost and appearance.

In our judgment and experience, there is not nearly enough emphasis placed on the proper selection and then careful monitoring, of appropriate electroacoustic characteristics for specific children. We are still, it seems, under the influence of research completed more than thirty years ago, which decried the concept of "selective amplification" and recommended instead one of two general patterns of amplification for all subjects (who, it should be noted, were adults with a normal background of language development, and not congenitally hearing-impaired children).

Our knowledge of the relationship between electroacoustic characteristics and speech intelligibility and our ability to modify these characteristics have increased tremendously since then; the clinical impact of this knowledge, however, is being imperfectly realized. That a child is wearing a perfectly functioning hearing aid is no reason to assume that the pattern of amplification it provides for him is also perfect, or as close to it as possible. That is to confuse a box (the hearing aid) with its contents (its electroacoustic characteristics). One would hardly accept the notion that a visually-impaired child could select at random satisfactory glasses from containers labelled "near-sightedness," "far-sightedness," "amblyopia," "astygmitism," and the like, but this is very often what we do when we select hearing aids and auditory trainers for hard of hearing children. We may not have the capability that optometrists have to prescribe precise, and appropriate, visual refractions, but we are not in the ear trumpet era either.

Unfortunately, we sometimes function as if we are. It is vital for any professional working with hearing-impaired children to have a working knowledge of the advantages and disadvantages of the general types of hearing aids suitable for children, the definition of the various electroacoustic characteristics, their implications regarding speech that is processed through a hearing aid, and the ability to meaningfully supervise their daily operation, that is troubleshooting.

Types of Hearing Aids There are four general types of personal hearing aids suitable for children: body aids, ear level aids, in-the-ear aids, and some member of the CROS family of hearing aids. We shall discuss each one briefly, indicating their advantages and disadvantages, and then comment on the merits of binaural amplification.

Body aids. These aids are considered to be sturdier than other types of hearing aids (though recent data on relative repair records are not available), and their controls are relatively easy for young children to manipulate. Because of their size, batteries last much longer in body aids than in other types of hearing aids. Feedback (high frequency whistle) is less of a problem with them, because of the greater distance between the microphone (located on the body) and the receiver—the "speaker" of the aid—at the ear. Less escaping sound from the receiver/mold combination is detected by the microphone, and since this escaping sound starts the feedback cycle that produces the audible squeal, the feedback cycle is less likely to occur. Above are perhaps the only current advangages of body aids over any other type. Since these aids are worn on the body, the speech signal is not detected at the normal ear level location. The microphone is frequently covered by layers of clothing, which muffles some high frequencies.

The influence of the body itself also produces some attenuation of important high frequencies and an enhancement of low frequencies. In other words, the high frequency amplification characteristics will be somewhat diminished and the low frequencies enhanced, relative to reported specification of the hearing aid. Moreover, body aids generally show poorer responses at the high frequencies than the newer generation of ear-level aids because these latter aids incorporate more efficient receivers. The rubbing of the microphone against the clothing whenever children are engaged in physical activity (and when are they not!) produces clothing noise—that is, audible sound that acts as both a masker and a distraction.

Body aids require that the nub of the transducer be snapped into the retaining ring of a standard earmold. This effectively precludes some of the manipulations of the earmold for possible advantageous acoustic effects (see discussion below). The use of binaural amplification is possible, but less physically convenient with body aids than with ear level aids. Except with infants and young children, we do not generally recommend body aids unless some specific set of circumstances, such as deformities of the pinna or ear canal, make it necessary to do so.

Ear Level Aids The type of ear level aid discussed here is the postauricular type, which fits behind the pinna, rather than eyeglass ear level aids, which are seldom used with children, and which are electroacoustically indistinguishable from postauricular aids.

Ear level aids incorporate all the electroacoustic possibilities found in body aids. But feedback can be much more of a problem with them because of the proximity of the microphone and the receiver (both located within the chassis of the aid). Battery life is relatively short, though much greater than it was years ago. The controls can be difficult for young children to manipulate, the internal settings are often so minute as to present a problem to the middle-aged audiologist with presbyopia (a magnifying glass is a good investment!). "Wind-noise" is a factor with many of them when they are worn outdoors on a windy day; an air turbulence is developed proximate to the microphone aperature and is perceived as a distracting and masking "hissing" noise. In our judgment, however, these disadvantages are outweighed by the advantages.

The aids are worn at ear level, the normal location for perceiving sounds. Directional/omnidirectional microphones are available (sometimes both in the same aid) so that the normal ear's azimuth detection capacities can be more closely replicated. A directional microphone, for example, will favor the detection of signals from a 45 degree arc in front of the child and suppress those arriving from the rear. Cosmetically, ear level aids are not only more acceptable to children, particularly the older ones, but they are often the only ones the children will countenance wearing. (We pay a penalty for this learned cosmetic focus when the children are required to wear the receiver packs of an FM auditory training device; they are often reluctant to do so in spite of the obvious acoustic advantages).

Earmold modifications of all kinds can be made, which frequently offers major acoustical advantages. Binaural units can be conveniently worn at ear level, with the normal interposition of the head (which carries with it desirable acoustical implications) between the two microphones.

In-The-Ear-Aids These aids are a relatively recent modification of post-auricular units. The entire aid, which includes the microphone, the electronic circuitry, the receiver, the battery, and various other controls, are inserted within the body of an earmold. This placement is the current ultimate in terms of normalizing the placement of the microphone and permitting the pinna to play their normal physiological role in sound reception. Contrary to some previous thought, the pinna are not just simply more-or-less ornamental appendages hung on the sides of our heads; they act as slight obstacles to high frequency sound reception from the rear and assist in the binaural reception and localization of speech (Preves and Griffing 1976).

Current models of in-the-ear aids include a wide range of fitting possibilities and, from an electroacoustic perspective, are perfectly suited for a wide range of moderate hearing losses. Currently they cannot be considered appropriate for young children because physical growth requires frequent replacement of their earmolds, the extraction and reinsertion of the aid into a new earmold, and because battery life is relatively short. These aids, however, can now be considered a viable alternative to postauricular ear level aids for hard of hearing adolescents with mild to moderate hearing losses.

CROS Hearing Aids Although not as recent as in-the-ear hearing aids, CROS hearing aids are also relative newcomers on the amplification scene. The acronym CROS stands for the Contralateral Routing of Offside Signals. The basic CROS is designed so that a microphone—inserted within an ear level hearing aid chassis—is placed behind a nonfunctional ear (or the "bad" ear). The signal from the microphone is directed via a wire connection, running under the hairline behind the neck to an amplifier/receiver placed in another ear level aid chassis behind the other (the "good") ear. This latter ear, the "good" ear, does not typically require amplification in its own right, although for optimal use there should be a mild, high frequency loss present in this ear.

The acoustic signal emanating from the receiver is coupled to this good ear via an open, or nonoccluding earmold, which thus does not impede the direct reception of speech going into the good ear. Only the signal reaching the microphone behind the bad ear is amplified. A CROS arrangement thereby enables a wearer to be aware and to respond to speech emanating from either side, although the signals from both sides are only heard in one "good" ear.

This is not, it should be emphasized, a binaural arrangement; it can best be characterized as a "V" connection with the tips of the "V" representing where sound is detected and the bottom tip of the "V" representing where the detected sound is directed. For some children, and in some situations, a CROS arrangement has been helpful, particularly where there is a need to respond to speech directed to the "bad" side. Some children, however, are confused by the arrangement; a supervised trial is best before making such a recommendation.

The other major member of the CROS family (there are others; audiologists have a penchant for devising fancy acronyms) is the BICROS, or the Bilateral Routing of Signals. For this arrangement, there is also one nonfunctional and one functional ear; the difference is that the functional ear (the "good" one) requires sound amplification in its own right. A microphone is placed behind the "bad" ear, as in the CROS aid, and the signals are again directed via a wire cord to the "good" ear; there is also, however, a complete ear level hearing aid including an open microphone behind the functional ear. Thus there are two microphones detecting acoustic signals, one behind each ear, but the sound they detect is transmitted to just one ear.

In a BICROS arrangement, the signals usually terminate in a closed mold otherwise feedback would be produced when the sound escaping from this ear is detected by the microphone and reamplified. In some instances, however, when the good ear exhibits a mild or moderate high frequency loss, it is possible to vent the earmold or to use a nonocculuding mold. In this circumstance, one would have to be sensitive to the possible production of feedback, and if it occurred, to modify the earmold. The basic advantage of the BICROS is the same as with the traditional CROS hearing aid— the child can receive, in his good ear, speech directed to either side of his head.

Binaural Hearing Aids We have already alluded to the provision of binaural hearing aids. Indeed, one of the advantages of ear level aids over body aids was the greater convenience in using binaural amplification. In our judgment—supported by the overwhelming preponderance of the evidence (see Ross 1980 for a review), binaural amplification is clearly the method of choice for most hearing-impaired children.

For some children, and their parents, there is a great deal of resistance to "putting another one of those things" on the ear; it is as if they will be considered, or consider themselves, doubly handicapped because they now wear two hearing aids. For others the cost may be prohibitive, although this should not be a major factor now given the mandate of many state agencies to provide such instruments (including possibly the public schools, with an IEP team recommendation). Still other children may not be audiological candidates for binaural amplification, those, for example, with a very wide disparity in hearing acuity or speech discrimination between their two ears; these are the children who may properly be CROS candidates.

Then there are some children whose apparent audiological suitability is not borne out even after an extensive trial with binaural amplification (and it *will* take time to determine a possible beneficial effect for older children with no prior experience with binaural amplified sound). In these instances, we may be seeing (and this is our personal conviction for the majority of such cases) the effect of binaural sensory deprivation. We make this point not just on the basis of our clinical experience and clinical intuition, but on the results of controlled animal research which clearly demonstrates binaural functional abnormalities after a period of monaural deprivation (Silverman and Clopton 1977; Clopton and Silverman 1977).

For the vast majority of hearing-impaired children, however, binaural hearing aids will improve their ability to comprehend speech, particularly in a noisy environment; it will make difficult listening situations less fatiguing; it will improve ability to localize the source of speech, which is very important in classroom discussions; and it will allow response with equal facility to speech directed to either ear. A bonus consideration is the fact that a binaural suprathreshold signal can produce the same loudness sensation as a monaural signal with 6 dB less SPL. If one is concerned with the possible deleterious effects of high sound pressure levels upon the impaired ear, this 6 dB reduction in the required output can be additonal protection for a child. We recommend that binaural amplification be the initial fitting of choice for all children unless definitely contraindicated by any of the examples given above. It is only when functioning with two aided ears is clearly poorer than (not equal to) functioning with one ear should one revert to monaural amplification.

electroacoustic modifications

Gain The gain of a hearing aid/auditory trainer is the difference between the input intensity (SPL) at the microphone and the output intensity (SPL) emanating from the transducer. Current—1976 ANSI (American National Standards Institute)—standards describe two basic methods of determining the gain. In one, the gain/volume control is turned to full-on and an input SPL of 60 dB (for aids without an automatic gain control) is delivered to the microphone. The 60 dB is subtracted from the average of the amplified output at 1000, 1600, and 2500 Hz to give the average full-on gain.

In the second method, the gain/volume control is set so that the output average, with the same 60 dB input at the three frequencies given above, is 17 dB below the saturation output of the hearing aid. This is called the reference test gain position and it is the gain setting used when evaluating the distortion and frequency response characteristics of a hearing aid. For example if the maximum possible output of a hearing aid averages 132 dB, then the output at the reference test gain position should average 115 dB or a reference test gain of 55 dB—that is, 115 dB minus 60 dB input. This setting is considered to be the standardized replication of the average gain setting that a person will or should use. One would not want to wear the aid with a full-on gain setting because of the increased likelihood of distortion in that setting. References therefore to the gain of a hearing aid without specifying whether it was measured with a full rotation of the gain control or in the reference test gain position, or some other possible method can be very misleading.

It is tempting to relate the gain of a hearing aid (by whatever method) to the degree of hearing loss a person manifests. So that if a child has a 60 dB hearing loss (SRT), it seems logical to amplifying speech by 60 dB, and thereby fully compensate for his hearing loss. Unfortunately, however, this is not how the ear operates. With a gain of 60 dB, and an input of 70 dB SPL, an output of 130 dB is produced (but see section on "Output" below for certain qualifications).

This figure is just about the average human tolerance for intense sounds (Morgan, Wilson, and Dirks 1974) and, in this example, is probably about 30 dB more gain than a person with this degree of loss would require. The so-called fifty-percent law for estimating gain states that the gain requirement of an individual is approximately one-half of the degree of his hearing loss—a gain of 30 dB for a 60 dB hearing loss.

A more refined rule of the thumb in estimating the required gain for a hearing-impaired person is to measure: 1) the SPL at various frequencies at which sound is comfortable (the MCL across frequencies), 2) note the SPL of an average intensity speech signal at these same frequencies, and 3) subtract the estimated input from the required output (the most comfortable point). In a later section of this chapter, we give several examples that elaborate on this concept.

What should be kept in mind here, however, is that it is not the degree of loss which is the primary determiner of the required gain of a hearing aid, but the output level required at each frequency subtracted from the usual input SPL's at the same frequencies. Since the gain required is a frequency dependent function (or a certain "frequency response," to be defined below), using a single gain figure to express a child's amplification needs can often be very deceptive. "Keeping it simple" is not always very "sound" advice.

Output   The electroacoustic dimension of output is often confused with gain. The output refers to the intensity of the amplified signal emitted by the hearing aid. In the example above, an input signal of 70 dB SPL and a gain of 60 dB, resulted in an output of 130 dB. It is this sound pressure which is delivered to the ear of a hearing-impaired person wearing a hearing aid.

The maximum power output (MPO) or the virtually indistinguishable SSPL 90 concept (Saturation Sound Pressure Level at 90 dB input) is the SPL at which no further increase is possible, regardless of input or gain. The SSPL 90 is measured by exposing a hearing aid, set on the full-on gain position, to a 90 dB SPL input across frequencies (from 200 to 5000 Hz at a minimum). The outputs at the frequencies 1000, 1600, and 2500 Hz are averaged to give the single figure defining the average SSPL 90 of the hearing aid. The maximum or peak SSPL 90 is the highest output occurring at any of the frequencies measured.

If the maximum SSPL 90 of a hearing aid is 130 dB, and the gain is set at 60 dB at that frequency, then an input of 70 dB results in an output of 130 dB. However, keeping the gain at 60 dB and increasing the input to 80 dB does *not* produce an output of 140 dB. The hearing aid cannot exceed its own limitations; the output remains at 130 dB.

What occurs for some types of hearing aids (those with output limited by "peak clipping") is an increase in distortion—that is, the fidelity of amplified signal is diminished. A reduction of the actual gain is a by-product of this type of overloading (like a cheap radio turned all the way up, the signal does not get louder, just more distorted). In other types of aids, those using an automatic volume control principle, the gain is automatically decreased or increased as the input is intensified or diminished; the usual distortion products are thereby minimized, although others may occur which relate to the time it takes for the gain to automatically increase and decrease. The point is, however, that no matter what method is used to limit the hearing aid's output, the maximum SSPL 90 cannot be exceeded.

An excessively high SSPL 90 is a very common reason why many hearing-impaired persons reject amplification. Satisfactory hearing aid usage cannot occur if the SSPL 90 exceeds a person's threshold of discomfort (TD). For example if a child's TD is 110 dB SPL, and the SSPL 90 of the hearing is 125 dB, he could tolerate inputs of 70 dB SPL with a gain of 40 dB, but any input greater than this would produce uncomfortable auditory sensations. Sounds of doors slamming, excessively loud speech, playground activities, cafeteria babble, dishes clashing, and heavy traffic would all probably produce input SPLs greater than 70 dB.

If such a child were to reduce the gain of his aid to keep the resulting outputs from exceeding his TD, he may not be able to understand speech delivered in an average intensity level. So he turns the gain up. Then, when he is again exposed to intense inputs, he reduces the gain. A few times like this, and the gain either stays reduced or the hearing aid stays out. The solution is to keep the gain at the required level, but to reduce the SSPL 90 to 110 dB.

The output of a hearing aid is the dimension of hearing aid performance which is often implicated regarding the possible effect of high sound levels upon the residual hearing. The question is often asked, if the SSPL 90 of a hearing aid is set too high, can this sound produce further decrements in hearing acuity? We know that the outputs of hearing aids and auditory trainers can exceed by far the SPL's which produce temporary or permanent threshold shifts for normally hearing individuals in occupational situations. Insofar as hard of hearing children are concerned, there are some grounds for caution, but not for alarm. Research has shown (Markides and Aryee 1978; Ross and Giolas 1978, for a recent review), that permanent shifts in auditory thresholds due to hearing aid trauma are a relatively rare, though real, phenomenon. Hearing aid outputs in excess of 132 dB SPL should be recommended only for those individuals with most severe hearing losses, as a precautionary measure.

An active audiology management program can detect possible problems as they occur, and before they become serious, and steps can be taken to alleviate the problem (such as reducing the output, switching a monaural aid from ear to ear, going from monaural to binaural amplification, and rolling off the low frequencies). Children should not be deprived of amplified sound, with all the implications sound has upon their communcation skills, academic performance, and behavioral adjustment, without serious thought to these consequences.

Frequency Response The frequency response of an acoustic device is an expression of its relative gain across frequency. A range of frequencies of precisely the same intensity is delivered to the microphone and because few if any hearing aids/auditory trainers can amplify such inputs to exactly the same degree, the output curve demonstrates different degrees of gain at the different frequencies. A so-called "flat curve" is the closest that can be achieved with current hearing aids to the theoretical equal amount of amplification at all frequencies—and in reality, this is not very "flat". A "high frequency" response is one which amplifies the high frequencies more than the lows. For conventional hearing aids, the ANSI 1976 standards require a 60 dB SPL input while the volume control is set to the "reference test gain" position (defined above).

Just about all hearing aids and auditory trainers include controls to adjust the frequency response to some extent. One can, for example, emphasize the low frequencies relative to the highs (occurring only rarely, when the person exhibits a rising threshold configuration) or the high frequencies relative to the lows (a common occurrance). Various degrees of selective amplification are possible. As with the gain, there is a temptation to compensate for the hearing loss by matching the frequency response to the hearing loss configuration. There are both problems and merit to this approach, but the preponderance of recent research increasingly supports the advantages of a modified form of a true "selective amplification" response (see Ross and Tommassetti 1979, for a general review of the literature).

The listening experience is a suprathreshold and not a threshold phenomenon. Our goal is to present to the children a pattern of amplified sound in a suprathreshold region which produces the greatest speech intelligibility or which is most comfortable (not necessarily the same pattern; the relationship between the two dimensions is still not clear).

The frequency response requirements at these suprathreshold listening levels cannot be predicted by generalizing from the threshold configuration only. For hearing-impaired persons who exhibit a gradually sloping threshold curve, there appears to be merit in duplicating the threshold configuration, with a hearing aid response, but not necessarily to the degree of loss at each frequency. That is, the person is provided with sufficient amplification at each frequency to produce an *aided* threshold curve which parallels, but does not equal, the normal *unaided* thresholds. Thus the person with a high frequency loss would receive relatively more amplification at the high frequencies than at the lows, in concordance to the actual degree of loss shown at the different frequencies (Pascoe 1975). For those with more extreme threshold slopes, it is the aided audibility area at the highest possible frequency bands (or the aided sensation level at these high bands) which is most closely related to speech perception (Skinner 1976).

This latter concept is in accord with our present concept of providing a child with the most—and *most salient*—acoustic information consistent with his hearing loss. The concept applies regardless of the slope and degree of loss. All we are saying here is that we want to maximize the amount of the important speech acoustic information that a child can receive with amplification, regardless of the type and degree of his hearing loss.

It is important to realize, however, that one cannot translate the frequency response specifications as they are published by a manufacturer to the actual sound pressures occurring in the ear canal of a specific child. The manufacturers follow ANSI 1976 standards, as they should, in making acoustic measurements of their instruments, and they use a standard 2 cc coupler as a real ear simulator. Real ears, however, particularly children's ears, vary to some degree or other from this "simulated" real ear (Villchur 1978). The difference between the cavity dimensions of an actual ear and the standard simulator, producing as it does differences in the SPL pattern existing in both cavities, is the reason we have emphasized measuring the functional frequency response of a hearing aid—that is the response obtained while the child is actually wearing the instrument.

Figure 4–4 gives an example of the wide variations from the coupler measured frequency response occurring in five normal ears (Dalsgaard and Jensen 1976). The solid line shows the results obtained in a 2 cc coupler, while the shaded area gives the real-ear variations. This figure shows how

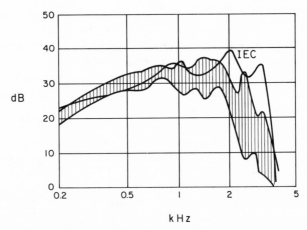

FIGURE 4-4 The difference between the 2 cc. coupler response of a hearing aid and the performance of the same aid (measured with a probe microphone in the ear) on five persons. The solid line represents the coupler response; the shaded area represents the individual real-ear variations (S. C. Dalsgaard and O. D. Jensen 1976. "Measurement of the Insertion Gain of Hearing Aids," *J. Audiol. Tech.* 15, 170. Reprinted by permission.

one cannot predict the electroacoustic performance of a hearing aid on a child simply by looking at the company's specifications.

Other evidence demonstrating this same effect is illustrated in Figure 4–5. In this figure the differences between the coupler and functional frequency responsed for ten hearing-impaired children are displayed across frequencies. The brackets indicate the wide standard deviations found among this group of children, who ranged in age from 7 to 10 years (Costa et al 1980).

Frequency Range Hearing aids and auditory trainers do not amplify extremely low and high frequencies. The frequency range refers to that band of frequencies that is effectively amplified by an instrument. In the ANSI 1976 method of determining the frequency range, the outputs at 1000, 1600, and 2500 Hz on the basic frequency response curve are averaged, and a horizontal line is drawn on the chart 20 dB below this average. The frequency range is defined as the points where this line intersects the upper and lower frequencies on the response curve.

A basic frequency response curve is displayed in Figure 4–6. The outputs at 1000, 1600, and 2500 Hz are 114, 110, and 109 dB, respectively, for an average of 111 dB. The horizontal line drawn 20 dB below, or at 91 dB, intersects the lower part of the curve at about 150 cps and the upper portion at about 5200 hz. This defines the frequency range of this instrument (the interested reader is referred to Pollack 1979 for a more precise description of this and all the other electroacoustic dimensions).

Frequency range is an extremely important, but frequently underestimated dimension of hearing aid performance, particularly as it applies to

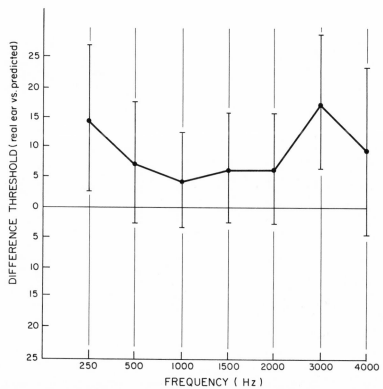

FIGURE 4–5 Means and standard deviations for the differences between the coupler and functional frequency responses. Ten hearing-impaired children, ranging in age from 7 to 14 years, were the subjects. The coupler responses predicted the gain would be greater than functional gain measures at each frequency.

congenitally hard of hearing children. Its significance can best be understood by relating it to the acoustics of speech signals, which are, after all, the signals we are most interested in amplifying for such children. As we have reviewed earlier, the vowels generally are of lower frequency and higher intensity than the consonants, with voiceless consonants showing the highest frequencies and some of the weakest intensities of any speech sounds.

The phoneme /s/, as Table 4–3 shows, is the consonant with the highest frequency components; it is also the one which carries the highest grammatical load. It is crucial, therefore, that the frequency range provided to children include sufficient low frequencies for vowel reception and sufficient high frequencies for unambiguous /s/ perception. Audiologists frequently express concern, and rightly so, about overamplifying the low frequencies because of the danger that high frequency perception will suffer due to an upward spread of masking—that is the intense low frequency components will render the high frequencies less audible. There is a difference, however

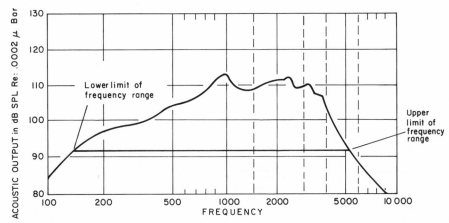

FIGURE 4–6 A base frequency response of a hearing aid used to compute the frequency range. The frequency response is obtained with a 60 dB input, and the aid is set at the reference test gain position. The frequency range is obtained by averaging the output at 100, 1600, and 2500 KHz, and drawing a horizontal line 20 dB below this average. The points where this line intersects the basic frequency response curves defines the upper and lower limits of the frequency range.

—as Daniel Ling has pointed out on innumerable occasions (personal communication)—between low frequency emphasis and low frequency extension. In the latter instance, the audibility of the vowels is ensured; they may be of less signficance than the consonants in regards to the comprehension of speech, but they are hardly useless. In the former instance, because of the spread of masking effects within the cochlea, the overamplification of the low frequency first formants may affect the person's ability to detect the rapid transitions of the higher frequency second formants.

Time and time again, as one observes the aided thresholds of children and relates them to the spectrum of speech and to the child's auditory thresholds in the high frequencies, it is apparent that many of the important high frequencies have been unnecessarily excluded from the child's awareness. There may have been some justification for this sorry situation some years ago, when the high frequency capability of hearing aids was limited, but this is not the case now.

Teachers of hard of hearing children and speech-language pathologists working with such children can attest to the efforts they expend in trying to teach, for example, the grammatical implications of the phoneme /s/; nearly an entire industry of structured language programs has evolved around this one problem alone. Yet this information is available in a natural, auditory fashion to many children for whom it is denied. Not only have advances in hearing aids made significant high frequency perception currently possible, but also some recent improvements in our knowledge about earmold acoustics, to which we shall now turn.

Earmold Acoustics   Earmolds have traditionally been thought of, at best, as just a conduit by means of which the sound emanating from the hearing aid receiver could be delivered into the ear canal and, at worst, simply a pain in the ear. In this section, we will summarize some of the acoustic effects made possible by modifying earmolds; as a matter of fact, much of the advances in the art of fitting hearing aids really refer to our increasing knowledge of earmold acoustics.

The simplest kind of earmold modification, referred to above in regards to CROS hearing aids, is to use no earmold at all, but simply to employ a frame to hold a section of tubing inserted into the ear (and in some cases, the frame itself can be dispensed with and just the tubing itself used). The acoustic effects of such an "open" condition, compared to a closed mold, is a reduction of the low frequency response below about 1000 Hz. At the same time, the direct reception of sound into the ear canal is unimpeded by an earmold, thus permitting the occurrence of the normal resonances in the external ear. These resonances are responsible for an increase in the sound pressure measured at the eardrum compared to the entrance at the canal of about 15 to 20 dB at the frequencies between 2000 and 7000 Hz—or a very significant amount of sound.

Venting an earmold is the most frequent type of modification employed. In the most common type of vent, a channel is drilled parallel to the channel delivering sound from the hearing aid through the earmold. This parallel bore thus by-passes the hearing aid and permits a direct air connection between the external atmosphere and the airpocket existing between the tip of the earmold and the eardrum.

The size of this vent, that is, its diameter, is what basically determines its acoustic effect. A very small vent will produce very little acoustical changes, but may serve to equalize the air pressure in the ear canal to the external air pressure. It thus may relieve a stuffy or uncomfortable feeling which sometimes occurs when a very tight earmold is used. Larger and larger vents begin to progressively diminish the low frequency response; the acoustic effect of the largest size vents approaches that of an "open" earmold.

Vent size can be used to fine tune the overall response of an electroacoustic system. Since the acoustical effect of a vent cannot easily be predicted in a real ear, since a child's need for a vent may vary with the situation—such as in quiet and noise—and since too large a vent may produce acoustic feedback at required gain settings, we recommend a valve (variable venting valve) or an insert (positive venting valve or select-a-vent), with which we can vary the diameter of the vent or close it entirely when necessary.

The diameter and length of a sound bore can be varied to change the electroacoustic characteristics impinging upon the eardrum. When the diameter of the sound bore is narrowed and its length increased, the low frequency response is enhanced, its range lowered, and overall sound pressure in the ear canal is increased. When the diameter of the sound bore is increased and its size diminished, a general shifting in the frequency response toward the high frequencies is noted. The interactions among these effects can be quite complicated, as many values of diameter and length can be selected. Some of these effects also work in opposition to one another, as when an earmold incorporates both a small and narrow diameter bore.

The difficulty in predicting the acoustic interactions of these modifications lend further support to the practice of measuring the aided response of hearing aids in a sound field. These measurements reflect the influence of all the factors, including earmolds, which modify the response of an electroacoustic system on a human being.

The last earmold modification to be discussed is the most recent and one that appears to be particularly beneficial for congenitally hard of hearing children. The cross-sectional diameter of the sound bore is progressively increased as it extends from the sound entry to the tip of the earmolds. This "step" or "horn" bore (the terminology has not yet been standardized) can considerably increase the high frequency range of an electroacoustic system (up to 7000 or 8000 Hz). Taken in conjunction with several acoustic filters inserted at proper points in the sound path from the receiver to the earmold, which depress unwanted peaks in the frequency response, it is possible to deliver to the eardrum a smooth, wide-band response of varying slopes of amplification (Killion 1978).

As a matter of fact, as often as possible we now recommend the step bore configuration for children, sometimes in conjunction with the acoustical filters and sometimes without them (depending on whether we want to retain or eliminate the hearing aid peak response at 1000 Hz). In brief, we now have a variety of ways to alter the real-ear response of a hearing aid using either the earmold or the aid itself.

troubleshooting hearing aids

There is no way we can take the continued operation and optimum performance of a hearing aid for granted (and we include here the receiver unit of an FM system, which functions also as a body worn hearing aid). These instruments, particularly as worn by children, exemplify a perfect instance of Murphy's law: if anything can go wrong, it will. We may have identified the acoustic correlates underlying the most salient speech perceptual clues; we may have provided the most effective amplification of the speech signal possible in an optimum acoustic environment; and we may have freely drawn upon the normal processes of speech perception in our expectations and training procedures; yet all of the preceding factors will be voided by a broken cord, a dead battery, or a poorly fitting earmold. If the auditory signal the child receives is distorted, intermittent, or frequently absent, if there is a random quality about auditory amplification, now it is here and now it is gone, now it is clear and now it is distorted, the child is likely to develop negative associations with the hearing aid. Moreover, he is likely to consciously or unconsciously focus his energies on the modality he can depend on: vision.

In our view, it may be preferable not to provide a hard of hearing child with amplification at all, than to supply him with a unit which is either inoperable or very distorted. We cannot then engage in the self-deceptive assurances that we are "doing all we can" in auditory management. If the child does not have amplification, then our deficiencies are apparent; we know what we must do. If he has amplification but it does not work or work well, and if this situation is not detected, it appears as if we are doing all we can for a child and the explanation for his poor or inconsistent performance is sought elsewhere—frequently by engaging in the "labeling" game— learning disability, does not pay attention, emotional problems. Until the child is old enough and skilled enough (and motivated enough) to trouble- shoot his own hearing aids, it must be done for him on a daily basis. Generally, it is considered the role of an IEP designate to troubleshoot the hearing aids, but regardless of who assumes the responsibility, it should be carried out at the beginning of every school day. Any questions that arise concerning the troubleshooting should be directed to the involved au- diology clinic, if the school is not fortunate enough in having a school-based audiologist.

Visual Inspection The first step is to look at the case for dents or other disfigurements. Although such occurrences by themselves do not indicate a concomitant electroacoustic problem, physical damage to the hearing aid is frequently associated with a malfunctioning instrument. The battery compartment should be opened and examined for corrosion and improper battery contact. Occasionally, one will find that the battery termi- nals are bent, corroded, or missing, resulting in an inadequate electrical connection. The batteries should be tested with a simple battery tester (the audiologist will know where this can be obtained) to see that they are registering the proper voltage, which is ordinarily 1.3 or 1.5 volts, and replacement batteries should be available.

The cords for body aids and CROS aids should be examined for the residue of chewing, twisting, or other hard knocks. Occasionally, the insula- tion may have been stripped from the cord, making a short circuit or a broken connection very likely. The cord prongs leading to and from the hearing aid and the receiver must fit snugly and be fully inserted.

A frequent cause for hearing aid malfunctions is damage to the receiver; it must manifest no cracks, dents, chewing gum, or other sequelae of hard treatment.

The tubing in ear level aids is examined for cracks, crimping and inflexi- bility. The tone hook (connecting the sound outlet from the aid to the

TABLE 4–7
Daily Visual Examination of Hearing Aid

PARTS	PROBLEMS	SOLUTIONS
Hearing aid case	Cracked	To dealer for repairs
Battery contacts	Corrosion, bent, or dirty	Clean with deoxide, tiny files, or erasor; straighten bent contacts
External controls (especially tone controls and telephone switch)	Not at correct settings	Adjust to recommended settings
Tone hook	Split or worn	Replace
Tubing or cords	Frayed, chewed, or worn	Replace
Cord prongs	Bent, improper connection	Replace entire cord
Microphone aperture	Covered with dust, food particles or other debris	Clean with small, short bristle brush; schedule electroacoustic analysis
Earmold bore	Occluded by cerumen	Rinse with mild detergent, clean with pipe cleaner.
Earmold	Loose or causes discomfort	New impression/mold
Batteries	Insufficient voltage (1.3 or 1.5)	New battery

tubing inserted in the earmold) must fit snugly at both ends. The external controls, for both body and ear level aids, must be verified for correctness each day. An aid set on the "T" (telephone) adjustment will not amplify sound. If an "H" (high-tone) adjustment is the recommended setting, "H" is what the aid should be set to.

The earmold is examined to determine if it is clean, intact, and unoccluded by cerumen. If it is dirty, it can be washed (minus the hearing aid, of course!) in warm water. Once inserted in a child's ear, the examiner observes whether it fits properly and does not result in acoustic feedback or discomfort. A summary of visual inspection factors are listed in Table 4–7.

Auditory (listening) Inspection The examiner listens to the aid with either his own earmold or a hearing aid stethoscope. This latter device permits listening to aids with an external receiver via a snap-on ring, or right through the earmold of either an ear level aid or a body aid, via a flexible connector into which the earmold is inserted (the audiologist should know where this can be obtained also). After some practice, the examiner should be able to determine if the aid sounds different than it had—that is if it is producing excessive distortion, noise, intermittent sounds, or inadequate amplification. This is a difficult experience for someone with normal hearing, because it may require listening to high level sounds; however, it is necessary because distortions may be apparent only at the high and not the low levels. A person with normal hearing should not be able to turn the volume all the way up and listen comfortably to an aid for a child with a severe hearing loss.

Checking the volume control is also important—that is, the signal should get louder gradually as the volume control is rotated rather than jump from little to maximum amplification with a slight increase in the control. When listening to body or CROS aids, the tester should manipulate the cords and listen to see if such manipulations produce static or an intermittent signal. If so, the cords should be replaced. A summary of listening examination checks are outline in Table 4–8.

TABLE 4–8

Daily Listening Examination

PROBLEM	POSSIBLE CAUSES	POSSIBLE CURES
No sound	Is on/off switch on?	Some switches operate with volume control; some aids have separate switches; some operate by opening and closing battery compartment
	Is battery OK?	Battery inserted; proper voltage; proper polarity; + and − orientation in battery compartment
	Is aid on "T"?	Telephone attachment bypasses microphone and detects electromagnetic signals only
	Is wire cord broken?	May not be apparent, because break occurs under insulation sheath; try a new cord
	Plastic tubing crimped shut?	This may block or severly reduce sound transmission.
	Cause not known	Return to dealer or factory
Intermittent sound	Short circuit in cord or volume control?	Manipulate cord; if intermittent, replace. Manipulate volume control; if intermittent, return to dealer or factory
	Poor battery contact?	Realign contacts
Poor sound quality	Weak battery?	Replace
	Is moisture or debris on diaphragm of microphone or receiver?	Clean and dry diaphragms; if no better return for repairs. Check electroacoustic analysis results
	Receiver malfunction?	Replace
	Microphone or circuitry malfunction?	Return to dealer or factory
	Unknown cause	Return to dealer or factory
Feedback	Poor fitting earmold? Increased middle ear impedance due to fluid or negative pressure	Check seating of mold; new earmold; otologic examination

Electroacoustic Analysis These daily visual/listening examinations must be supplemented by frequent electroacoustic analysis. Relatively low cost devices are now available in many audiology programs to accomplish this task. We have already, in the evaluation section, suggested the specific dimensions which should be included in such an analysis.

We recommend that they be conducted routinely two or three times a year and on such occasions when the results of the visual/listening examinations suggest a need. Basically, we want to verify that the instrument is functioning as recommended and as it has been previously. No one now questions the need for the frequent monitoring of a child's hearing, particularly when possible problems are evident; the electroacoustic product of hearing aids are likely to show much greater variations over time than a child's hearing, and consequently must be monitored that much more. The stability of their performance simply cannot be taken for granted, certainly not when they are worn by children.

aided residual hearing

The three preceding factors interact with a child's hearing loss to produce the acoustic goal of our efforts: aided residual hearing. In determining the target output which maximizes aided residual hearing, we should also consider a factor not heretofore mentioned, and that is the perceived spectrum of speech occurring in a normal ear. This is not as obvious as it may seem.

In arriving at the pattern of speech *sensation* levels occurring in a normal ear, one has to consider the interactions of the usual speech spectrum (Figure 4–2), the normal threshold configuration across frequency (relatively poor sensitivity at the lower frequencies), and the acoustic effect of the head, pinna, and ear canal upon the speech sound pressures occurring at the eardrum. From an evolutionary standpoint, the acoustic product of speech production and the anatomical structures designed to receive this product have been superbly adapted to one another. This serves to optimize the acoustic transmission of information between people.

We should not, when amplifying speech, disrupt the normally perceived speech spectrum more than we have to. Although it is obvious that a hearing loss will reduce the absolute sensation levels of speech for a hearing-impaired listener, we can still try to replicate, as far as we can, the pattern of speech sensation levels (the frequency response, if you will) which occurs in the normal listener.

The average speech sensation levels across frequency for 20 normal listeners is given in Figure 4–7 (adapted from Pascoe 1978). Note that the normal sensation level of speech is not a smooth continuous function. Rather, the highest sensation levels of speech occur in two frequency re-

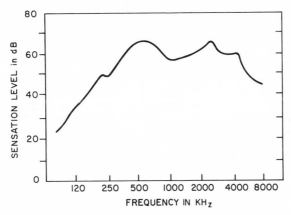

FIGURE 4–7 The perceived spectrum of speech in a normal ear. The speech spectrum is modified by the head, pinna and ear canal, and the threshold frequency response of the normal ear to produce the sensation levels indicated in the illustration.

gions, a low one centered at 630 Hz and a high one at 2500 Hz. The two peaks differ by no more than 3 dB, while the sensation level at 1000 Hz is 8 dB lower than the peaks. It has been hypothesized that this total effect contributes to the audibility of friction sounds, as well as to the detection of second formant transitions (Miller 1973).

The dip at 1000 Hz is a particularly interesting finding, in view of the usual emphasis in the response of hearing aids at this frequency. If we reflect upon how the normal ear modifies the speech spectrum, and it would be unwise to simply view this as an evolutionary accident, it is obvious that hearing aids have been emphasizing a frequency region which should have been deemphasized.

One of our major goals as we view the pattern of aided residual hearing occurring in a specific child is to ensure that this does not happen. In attempting to replicate this pattern as much as possible for a child with a severe hearing loss, we would, however, view with caution the peak at 630 Hz. The impaired cochlea exposed to high sound pressures may produce a spread of masking effects and interfere with the discrimination of the vital second format transitions. Nevertheless, this normative information can serve as the basis from which we can view the aided pattern of residual hearing for hard of hearing children.

The only current clinically feasible method we have for assessing the aided sensation levels of speech for a hard of hearing child is the use of aided, sound-field audiometry.* In this test the child is seated about three

---

*We would hope, however, as we stated earlier, that this situation will soon change as more clinical programs adopt the ear-canal microphone method for measuring the sound pressures existing in an ear canal as a result of hearing aid amplification (Harford 1980).

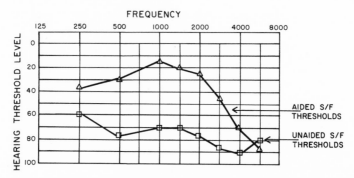

FIGURE 4–8 Conventionally plotted aided verses unaided sound field measures. A calibrated sound field is required to relate the obtained thresholds to those obtained with ear phones.

feet from a loudspeaker in an audiometric test suite and he is required to respond to warble tones or narrow band noises emanating from the speaker. In the most commonly employed procedure, the unaided and aided sound-field thresholds are plotted on a typical audiogram. A typical example of an audiogram with unaided and aided sound-field thresholds is given in Figure 4–8. Such a plot can graphically display the functional gain and frequency response of a hearing aid (the difference between the aided and the unaided thresholds across frequency).

The relative differences occurring between various types of aids, adjustments, and earmolds can be plotted, and thus make the electroacoustic distinctions between them very evident.

Some audiologists use this graphic presentation of aided and unaided thresholds to demonstrate to parents and other professionals how "normal" the child's hearing has become with amplification. In trying to convey this idea, one has to be very careful to distinguish between the degree of help (amplification) provided by the hearing aid, and viewing the aided threshold configuration as being equivalent to an unaided hearing loss of the same extent.

Aided listening is not the same as unaided listening, even though the absolute sound-field thresholds in both conditions are the same (assuming a calibrated sound-field). For one, in the aided condition, a much higher SPL actually reaches the cochlea than in the unaided condition (speech input plus hearing aid *gain* equals output). The ear, particularly the damaged ear, does not function the same at high sound-pressure levels as a more normal ear would at lower SPLs. For another, the hearing aid itself produces distortions, which may interact with the distortions occurring in the ear itself, to further distinguish between aided and unaided listening (Table 4–6 shows how aided listening can diminish speech perception scores compared to unaided listening).

Plotting the aided versus the unaided threshold configuration on an audiogram does not conveniently lend itself to an analysis of the aided

154

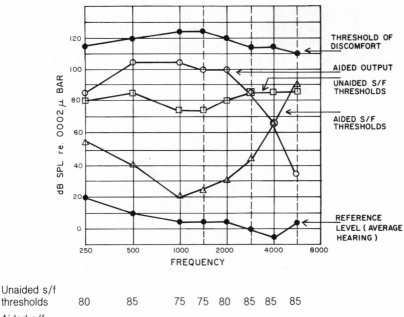

Unaided s/f thresholds	80	85	75	75	80	85	85	85
Aided s/f thresholds	55	40	20	25	30	45	65	90
Gain	25	45	55	50	50	40	20	-5
Speech input	60	60	50	50	50	45	45	40
Aided output	85	105	105	100	100	85	65	35
Threshold of discomfort	115	120	125	125	120	115	115	110

FIGURE 4–9 Sound field results of the previous example (Figure 4–9) plotted with an SPL scale. Plotting the results in this fashion permits a more detailed analysis of the child's aided residual hearing.

residual hearing. One has to understand that an aided audiogram is a *threshold* configuration; the sound intensity emanating from the sound-field loud-speaker is increased until the child responds. This is not what normally happens in real life.

In a reality situation, the child is exposed to a speech spectrum input of some 60 to 70 SPL that is increased by the gain of the hearing aid and results in a *suprathreshold* listening experience. We should have some way of looking at the output characteristics of a hearing aid to a normal speech spectrum input, plotted in relation to a child's hearing loss. There are advantages of plotting these and all the other relevent dimensions of hearing aid performance and hearing loss on an SPL scale rather than an HTL scale as in Figure 4–8. We can, thereby, refer all of our measures and computations to the same reference level and thus obtain a clear graphic portrayal of the child's residual hearing. Let us consider several examples.

For our first one, note the aided audiogram in the previous figure, but this time plotted on an SPL scale with the other dimensions of interest

155

included on the same chart (Figure 4–9). (At this point, we would ask some of our readers not to consider the concepts we will be discussing as just in the province of the audiologist, and dismiss them as being too "technical" for speech-language pathologists and teachers of hearing-impaired children. These concepts deal with aided residual hearing, the product of our efforts to date, and thus directly concern the educational responsibilities of all professionals vis à vis their hearing-impaired children.)

In an SPL chart, increasing intensity is depicted as rising from the bottom of the ordinate, unlike an audiogram in which increasing hearing loss (and thus increasing intensity) descends from the top to the bottom. The reference sound-field thresholds on the bottom of Figure 4–9 approximates (to the nearest 5 dB, to simplify clinical measurements) the unaided, monaural, sound-field thresholds which would be obtained on normally hearing listeners (Morgan, Dirks, and Bower 1979). The SPLs representing the "average" threshold are less than are found with earphones (ANSI 1969). This difference reflects the different conditions of listening, earphone versus sound field. (To simplify clinical measurements, it may be possible to employ these predictable differences as corrections to earphone measured thresholds of hearing, and plot the resulting values directly on an SPL chart, assuming, of course, a calibrated sound field. For example, if at 4000 Hz, sound-field thresholds were normally 10 dB better than earphone thresholds, all one would have to do is deduct 10 dB from the earphone measurements and plot the number on the SPL sound field audiogram.)

The hearing loss depicted in Figure 4–9 is the same as the one shown in Figure 4–8. Note the unaided sound-field threshold curve in respect to the reference levels; at 250 Hz, it is 60 dB above the reference; at 500 Hz, it is 75 dB above; at 1000 Hz it is 70 dB above; and so on. These are exactly the hearing levels shown on the conventional sound field audiogram. We have simply turned it upside down.

The aided sound-field thresholds, also taken from Figure 4–8, are similarly reversed; they show the improvement in the absolute thresholds as a function of amplification. The SPL values of the unaided and aided sound-field thresholds are given in the first two rows of numbers on the figure. The advantages of this plot should now (we hope) become evident, as we consider other dimensions underlying aided residual hearing.

The third row of numbers represents the functional gain of the hearing aid, or the difference between the aided and the unaided performance across frequency. The fourth row is an approximation of the SPL in a speech signal at the indicated frequencies (Pascoe 1978). These figures serve as an input estimate that, when added to the gain in the previous row, give us the aided output of the hearing aid.

The parameter labeled "aided output" on the figure now displays the relationship between this curve and the unaided threshold curve. *The area between them is the aided residual hearing. This is the sound pattern the child detects with a hearing aid.* We are able to make this observation because both parameters have been plotted with the same reference level.

One more parameter should be discussed before we analyze the aided residual hearing (which can, and is, also termed the aided pattern of sensation levels across frequency). This last one is the threshold of discomfort. The last row of numbers gives the values of the TD, which is also plotted as the topmost curve on the figure. The difference between the aided output and the TD is the "reserve" available when the gain is increased beyond the indicated levels, or when the child is exposed to more intense inputs (but keep in mind that a speech signal includes peak energies about 12 dB higher than the specific warble tone, or narrow band output levels given here). The SPLs of the TD also define the limits which should not be exceeded with the SSPL 90 (in Ross and Tommassetti 1979, and Hawkins 1980, a method is given whereby real ear SPL TDs can be converted to coupler defined SSPL 90s, thus enabling an audiologist to reconcile the different reference levels of these two measures).

Now let us analyze the aided residual hearing area as it is displayed in Figure 4–9. We emphasize that in arriving at this value, we have used an estimate of real speech spectrum input, and measured the performance of the entire electroacoustic system as it is worn by a child. Although we cannot claim psycho-acoustic exactitude in arriving at this goal, we can assert that what we have plotted is the best approximation we can achieve at the present state of the art.

Keeping in mind the pattern of desired sensation levels given in Figure 4–7, we can see that this hearing aid provides insufficient amplification at the high frequencies and too much gain at 1000 Hz. This child can detect speech signals adequately to about 2000 Hz, and thus the second formants of male voices are available to him, but he will have some difficulty perceiving the second formants of the front vowels as spoken by women and children (Table 4–1). He can hear the lower portion of the /sh/, but he will have a problem detecting the rest of the fricatives, particularly the voiceless ones.

The burst energy of the voiceless plosives fall beyond the limits of his aided residual hearing, though he can use the second formant transitions of most of the vowels as an effective perceptual clue. With this kind of aided residual hearing pattern, this child should not do too badly, but we can do a lot better for him (let us not be satisfied with just some help). Consider the next figure, where we have modifed the response of the same hearing aid for a more desirable pattern of sensation levels (Figure 4–10).

Note that we have increased the gain slightly at 250 Hz, decreased it at 500, 1000, and 1500 Hz, and substantially increased it again at 3000 Hz and beyond. The resulting aided residual hearing pattern is fairly equal across frequencies. We have reduced the peak at 1000 Hz, and extended the frequency range sufficiently to encompass the sibilants of speech.

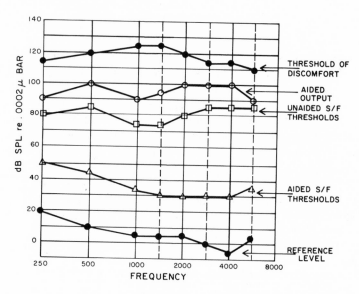

Unaided s/f thresholds	80	85	75	75	80	85	85	85
Aided s/f thresholds	50	45	35	30	30	30	30	35
Gain	30	40	40	45	50	55	55	50
Speech input	60	60	50	50	50	45	45	40
Aided output		100	90	95	100	100	100	90
Threshold of discomfort	115	120	125	125	120	115	115	110

FIGURE 4–10 Modification of the frequency response plotted in Figure 4–9 to produce a more desirable pattern of aided residual hearing.

To do this we have increased the gain of the aid to the practical limits of an ear-level instrument. Although more gain is technically feasible, and is possible in some cases, acoustic squeal is a real danger with any more gain. Note, too, that the aided threshold curve closely parallels the normal threshold curve, a goal we referred to earlier, and that there is some, albeit limited, "head room" between the aided output and the TD. This permits some more increased inputs without exceeding the TD. This is an example of a child with a severe hearing loss, and the range between the aided output and the TD is not so great as we would like. In such cases, the use of a hearing aid incorporating an automatic gain control (a compression hearing aid) feature could be considered. If we could obtain the results shown in Figure 4–10, however, for such a child, we would have reason to feel moderately content with our efforts.

At the present state of the art, it would be desirable to confirm our electroacoustic recommendations and findings with speech audiometry, whenever possible. There are dimensions of hearing aid performance, such

158

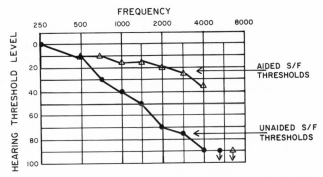

FIGURE 4-11 An example of a conventionally plotted unaided versus aided audiogram for a child with a high-frequency loss.

as various kinds of distortions, which this procedure does not take into account. For this reason, and because we lack definitive research into an unknown number of variables and details, we still require confirmation of the "aided residual hearing" concept. The basic procedure, however, is a logical extension of our present knowledge and where the future lies. Indeed some investigators have already related what is in essence aided residual hearing to speech intelligibility and found higher relationships than with any other measure of electroacoustic performance (Studebaker and Wark 1980; Dugal et al 1980). The clinical application of this concept may be a long time arriving, and in the meantime we have to deal with children with the best knowledge we have. We should also note that speech audiometry, particularly as practiced with children, is fraught with many known variables and is in itself a crude but sometimes useful, tool for selecting an appropriate electroacoustic system.

In this next, and last, example, we shall consider the aided residual hearing area for a child with a moderate high frequency hearing loss. Children with losses of this degree and type are probably more frequently found in the public schools than that given in the previous example. The unaided and aided thresholds are plotted in Figure 4-11, and on an SPL audiogram in Figure 4-12. Note again in the SPL chart that the range between the aided output and the unaided sound-field threshold defines the goal of our efforts, the aided residual hearing (or the aided sensation level) across frequency.

This is a child whose unaided residual hearing extends only to 4000 Hz, and for whom we have endeavored to ensure an adequate aided sensation level up to this point. As in the previous example, we would have liked to provide more gain at 4000 Hz, but are limited by the dangers of incurring acoustic feedback.

We must consider the possibility that such a child, who has not previously worn hearing aids, or whose first aid did not produce the high frequency emphasis evident here, would find this pattern of aided residual hearing uncomfortable and would reject amplification. In our judgment, if the con-

159

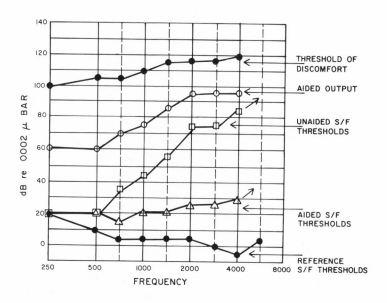

Unaided s/f
thresholds 20   20 35 45 55 75 75 85 NR

Aided s/f
thresholds 20   20 15 20 20 25 25 30 NR

Gain   0   0   20 25 35 50 50 55 –

Speech input 60 60 50 50 50 45 45 40 –

Aided output 60 60 70 75 85 95 95 95

Threshold of
discomfort 100   105 105 110 115 115 115 120

FIGURE 4–12 The same sound field results as in the previous example, but plotted on an SPL scale. The residual hearing range is the difference between the unaided sound field thresholds and the aided output. The numerical values of the indicated parameters are given in the rows of numbers.

cept of "auditory training" has any validity at all for congenitally hard of hearing children—and we think it does—it must be applied in such instances. Of course, a child (and adults, too, for that matter) who has only experienced auditory sensations in the low and middle frequencies may find this degree of high frequency emphasis uncomfortable.

Having no previous exposure to high frequency sound, not yet able to associate the acoustic information to its linguistic counterpart, or unable to integrate the new signals with his old familiar patterns, certainly this child may well find the experience disconcerting and unpleasant. For a while, he may even show a diminished capacity to comprehend speech. What he requires is a graduated series of approximations. Each one closer to the final, and theoretically ideal goal, until he can integrate and use the new auditory sensations to enhance his speech perception capacity.

It may be that he will never be able to effectively exploit the high frequencies; considering the potential value of the additional acoustic information, however, the attempt must be made. This is what the therapeutic process is all about. We do not view our goal of maximizing the residual hearing capacity as occurring, or being possible, in one or two "hearing aid evaluation" encounters. We do view this goal as being the product of a number of ongoing therapeutic visits, with each one devoted to the exploration of various electroacoustic possibilities—keeping in mind the ideal pattern of aided sensation levels and the need to constantly verify our recommendations with behavioral observations.

For a child with this degree of high frequency hearing loss, the concept of auditory sensory deprivation applies, though in a limited fashion. If such a child has never been exposed to the high frequency unaided bands of speech, and the degree of his loss precludes unaided exposure to these frequencies, then the auditory neurons and structures associated with them will not have experienced the auditory stimulation necessary for optimum development. Granted that this postulated "band-limited" sensory deprivation has not been confirmed experimentally, but why take chances? If the child does demonstrate potentially usable residual hearing in the high frequencies, we are obligated to make it available to him, and that means precluding the possible physiological effects consequent to a localized, band-limited auditory sensory deprivation. Early and appropriate amplification is the answer to this problem.

FM auditory trainers: description, selection, utilization

Given even a moderately acceptable aided residual hearing pattern, the single most important determiner of speech perception through an electroacoustic system is the relationship between the intensities of the speaker's voice and the noise level existing at the microphone. If the speech signal is buried in the noise, no amount of other considerations is going to make that signal intelligible. The greater the degree the speech signal exceeds the noise (that is, the higher the signal to noise ratio), the more intelligible the speech signal will become. This function levels off for hearing-impaired individuals at a sensation level of 33 dB for consonants and 22 dB for vowels (Gengel, in Stark 1974, p. 131) or at about an overall signal to noise ratio of 25 to 30 dB.

The main purpose, and major attribute of an FM auditory training system, is to enhance the signal to noise ratio, and thus help create the acoustic conditions for maximizing speech perception. This enhancement is a consequence of exploiting the concept illustrated in Figure 4–3. In brief, by locating the microphone of the auditory trainer close to the speaker's mouth, the intensity of the speech signal is augmented relative to the ambient noise levels. Actually, of course, the effect will occur with any kind of

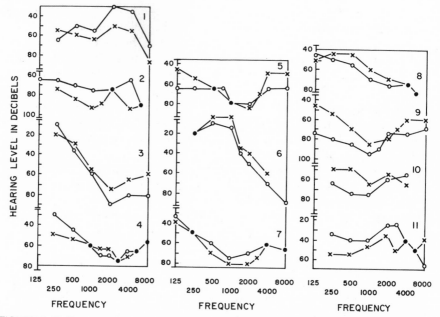

FIGURE 4–13 Pure-tone threshold audiograms of eleven hard of hearing children whose speech discrimination scores were tested in an ordinary classroom under FM and no FM conditions (results given in Table 4–9).

electroacoustic system (hearing aids, hard-wire auditory trainers) as long as the microphone positioning is favorable (Ross 1978).

We stress, as indicated above, the FM wireless auditory trainer to capture this effect in regular classrooms because it is the only such device currently available that will permit this advantage in such settings. There is no way that we can assert with enough vigor how crucial the provision of such devices can be for hard of hearing youngsters being educated in our educational mainstream. We personally know of many instances where it has made the difference between educational success and educational failure.

For example, consider the eleven hard of hearing children whose air conduction pure-tone thresholds are given in Figure 4–13. Their speech discrimination scores were measured in an ordinary classroom, at a distance between 8 and 14 feet from the talker, with an FM auditory trainer and with their usual amplification condition (Ross, Giolas, and Carver 1973). The results are given in Table 4–9. The differences are apparent, sometimes dramatically so—ranging from a minimum inprovement of 12% to a maximum of 76%! Nine of these eleven children had been tested in a similar study three years previously, with very similar results (Ross and Giolas 1971).

Consider the scores once again. Note how poorly the children understood speech under their usual amplification condition and the magnitude of the improvement with an FM system. Is it possible to think of any other

162

TABLE 4-9
Word Discrimination Scores Obtained with Eleven Hard of Hearing Youngsters
While Receiving an FM Transmitted Speech Signal and While Wearing
Their Usual Amplification Device (binaural, monaural, or none)

Nine of these children were tested three years previously with similar results

SUBJECT	FM AUDITORY TRAINER	USUAL AMPLIFICATION CONDITION*	DIFFERENCE
1	48	20 (M)	28
2	98	52 (M)	46
3	24	12 (M)	12
4	68	16 (M)	52
5	22	8 (B)	14
6	58	36 (N)	22
7	50	30 (B)	20
8	24	4 (B)	20
9	52	16 (B)	36
10	98	22 (B)	76
11	96	26 (N)	70
Mean	58	22	36

*M = Monaural; B = Binaural; N = None

kind of remedial measure which can be applied to hard of hearing children which can pay greater, more immediate dividends? Somehow its very simplicity militates against its acceptance; it is as if we can only accept those improvements in children's functioning which require great expenditures of energy (not to mention blood, sweat, and tears!).*

Description An FM wireless auditory training system consists of a microphone/transmitter worn by the teacher and an FM receiver/hearing aid worn by the child, and, except for battery rechargers, that is all there is. There are no wire loops around the room or earphones which have to be plugged into a fixed location. The microphone is normally suspended around the teacher's neck, thereby ensuring the favorable talker-microphone distances responsible for the resulting good signal to noise ratio. The transmitters, which ordinarily broadcast in the 72s to 76 MHz band, are permitted sufficient transmitting power by FCC regulations to virtually guarantee an equal distribution of signal strength within the confines of even large classrooms (in other words, no "dead" spots which may occur with other kinds of systems).

There are 32 carrier-wave frequencies within the band, thus obviating possible interference from nearby transmitters on the same frequency. If

---

*New developments are adopted at a snail's pace. This is evident from the date of these references. The first study was reported ten years ago. One wonders just how many hard of hearing children have been under or maleducated in the ensuing years at the same time, a therapeutic tool has been available which could significantly reduce the extent of these children's school-based problems. We firmly believe that most educators and administrators have the best of intentions; unfortunately, this is not always accompanied by effectiveness of information. As we mentioned before, time is not on our side when we work with children, and we trust that the next ten years will see more children using FM systems appropriately in classrooms.

interference occurs, it is a simple matter to select another carrier-wave frequency. The children's receivers (not a hearing aid transducer, which is also termed a "receiver", but the device which detects or "receives" the FM signal) are tuned to the required frequency, either with plug-in modules or with a two-position selection switch.

One (monaural) or two (binaural) environmental microphones are included with FM receiver units, permitting them to also serve as body monaural or binaural hearing aids when the FM transmission is not appropriate. These microphones enable the children to monitor their own vocal output and to directly hear the other children.

Most FM auditory trainers are powered by rechargeable energy cells. Essentially, the system can be conceptualized as no more than an FM radio, with the teacher "broadcasting" a signal which the child detects on his own "radio."

Four representative makes of currently available FM auditory training systems are shown in the following figures. In Figure 4–14, the device is displayed in a five-unit recharger. The numbers on the microphone and the receiver are transmission frequencies; this model permits the selection of one of two transmitting and receiving frequencies.

A slightly different arrangement is shown in Figure 4–15. In this model, the microphone and transmitter are separated; the transmitter is worn on the teacher's belt, while the microphone is positioned via a velcro fastener on the upper torso.

Still another kind of arrangement is shown in Figure 4–16. The transmitter is in the middle, made to be worn around the teacher's neck. The right hand unit converts the speech signal to a magnetic field via the loop which is worn around the child's neck. This signal is converted to an electrical signal by the telephone coil of a postauricular hearing aid. An environmental microphone on the receiver permits child-to-child communication and

FIGURE 4–14 FM auditory training unit in a five-unit battery recharger. (Courtesy of Biocoustics, Inc.)

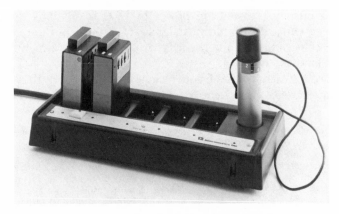

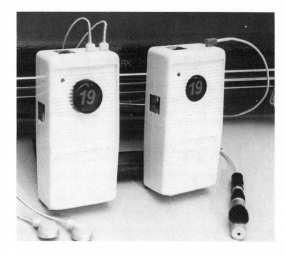

FIGURE 4–15 FM microphone/ transmitter and receiver. The microphone and transmitter are separate units. (Courtesy of Earmark, Inc.)

self-monitoring. The left-hand unit is designed to operate with a personal hearing aid, via a direct wire connection from the FM receiver to the aid. When the FM receiver is not needed, or at home, the cord can easily be disconnected.

A close-up view of a stereo receiver is shown in Figure 4–17. As indicated, the unit permits a great deal of electroacoustic modifications to be made to each ear separately.

FIGURE 4–16 FM auditory training system with two types of receiver. The center unit is the microphone. The right-hand unit is a receiver with an induction coil output; the loop is placed around the child's neck and the resulting electromagnetic field is picked up by the child's hearing aid set on the telephone or microphone/telephone position. The output from the receiver on the left connects to a personal hearing aid via a wire cord. (Courtesy of HC Electronics, Inc.)

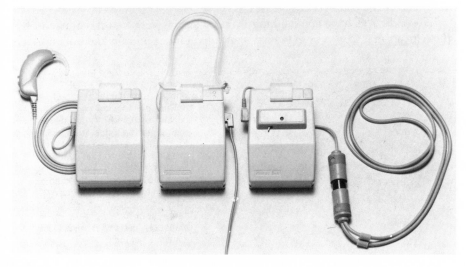

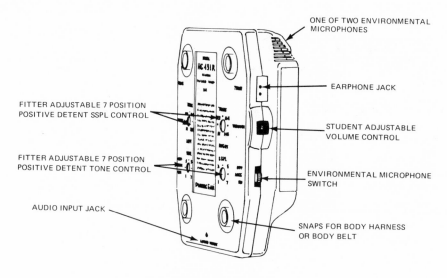

ONE OF TWO ENVIRONMENTAL MICROPHONES

EARPHONE JACK

FITTER ADJUSTABLE 7 POSITION POSITIVE DETENT SSPL CONTROL

STUDENT ADJUSTABLE VOLUME CONTROL

FITTER ADJUSTABLE 7 POSITION POSITIVE DETENT TONE CONTROL

ENVIRONMENTAL MICROPHONE SWITCH

AUDIO INPUT JACK

SNAPS FOR BODY HARNESS OR BODY BELT

HC 431R FM PHONIC EAR   STEREO STUDENT RECEIVER WITH MULTI-VARIABLE FITTING CAPABILITIES

FIGURE 4–17 A close-up view of an FM receiver that incorporates binaural microphones for the reception of environmental signals. (Courtesy of HC Electronics, Inc.)

In Figure 4–18, the microphone and the speaker (the hearing aid receiver) are both located in the housing of a postauricular hearing aid. The auditory signals are detected at ear level, referred back to the receiver pack on the body for electroacoustic processing, and rereferred back to the ear-level aid. This arrangement permits the additional control over an acoustic signal which modifications in earmolds can produce. The FM signal is received by the body unit and the signal is routed to the ear-level transducers. This unit is also made to be used with either rechargeable or disposable batteries as shown in Figure 4–19.

These devices have come a long way since they were first introduced on the educational scene about twelve years ago. They generally did not, at that

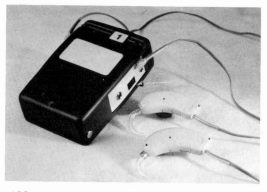

FIGURE 4–18 An FM receiver in which the environmental microphones and the hearing aid receivers are located at ear level; signals detected by the environmental microphones are shunted to the body unit where they are directed back to the ear-level hearing aid transducers (receivers). The FM signal is detected by the FM receiver located in the body unit and delivered to the same transducers in the usual manner. (Courtesy of Telex Communications, Inc.)

166

time, permit the choice of varying electroacoustic possibilities, and their performance stability and repair record can only be termed abysmal. More often than not, some component of the unit (the microphone, transmitter, FM receiver, or environmental microphones) would not operate at all, or would function very poorly. Teachers, children, and everyone involved would simply get discouraged and revert to using hearing aids, in spite of the occasionally successful use and apparent benefit of the FM instrument. Their performance stability is much better now—though still in need of improvement—and back-up units are available when the devices are inoperable or are being repaired.

Recommended Features   In the paragraphs to follow, we shall list and describe some of the recommended features to be found in current FM wireless auditory training systems. Not all of them are incorporated in every manufacturer's unit, and not all are equally desirable. Since research support is lacking for many of the features, we are defining a "desirable" feature on the basis of our own judgment and experience. Also, the order in which they appear below is no indication of their relative importance; except for possibly the first one, we simply have no basis for making this distinction.

(1) All FM systems that we are aware of incorporate controls for modifying the frequency response and the ouput of the receiver unit. This is an essential provision in all such instruments, permitting variations

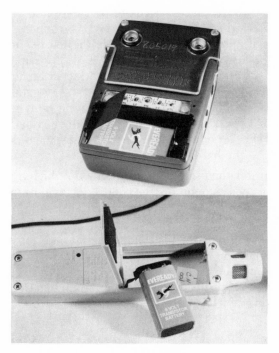

FIGURE 4–19 A close-up view of an FM microphone/transmitter and receiver that can utilize either rechargeable or disposable batteries. (Courtesy of Telex Communications, Inc.)

in the electroacoustic characteristics to suit individual requirements. The modifications are such that the output can be reduced to accommodate the mildest hearing loss, and frequency response can be adjusted to suit most hearing loss configurations. In binaural units, each channel can be set separately, for the child who does not have the same hearing loss in both ears.

(2) A number of systems include a provision for routing the output of the FM receiver through personal postauricular hearing aids, rather than the snap-on transducers. The hearing aids function as they ordinarily would, but they also process the FM transmitted signal. The children wear their own hearing aids (which have been properly adapted) to school, attach the FM unit to the aids, and remove it when it is time to go home.

(3) We think it is desirable for FM devices to include binaural reception of environmental signals. This is not an issue when the focus is on the teacher's speech, but it very well may be during periods when it is not appropriate to employ the teacher's microphone—for example, during lunch. At such times, the child's unit is used like a hearing aid and in most cases should be binaural.

(4) It is sometimes useful for the teacher's microphone to include the capability of receiving an auxiliary input, such as from a tape recorder, sound movie projector, or television monitor. These devices often emit noise while they are operating, which would be picked up by an acoustic coupling of the microphone to the sound source.

An auxiliary input permits a direct electrical connection between the teacher microphone and the sound source. And some FM microphone/ transmitters include an optional talkover circuit to enable the teacher to override the auxiliary input for instructional purposes. It is also possible with some systems to make a direct electrical connection with an auxiliary input to the child's receiver. Problems may arise when using the auxiliary input if the sound source is not capable of accommodating both an auxiliary output and an external speaker. That is, the use of the auxiliary circuit deactivates the external speaker of the source. In such cases, the only one to hear the sound would be the hard of hearing child.

(5) Several FM systems allow for the use of an induction loop which the child wears around his neck. In such a condition, the child's personal hearing aids are used in the telecoil mode and the FM signal is transmitted to the loop, converted to a magnetic field, and delivered to the hearing aids through the telecoil. In order for this to work, the child's personal aids must either have a telecoil or be modified to have one. Several problems arise in this arrangement stemming from the lack of manufacturer's specifications for the telecoil, therefore, one does not know if the output and frequency response of the hearing aid microphone are the same with the telecoil.

The receiver that the child wears must also have an environmental micro-phone on it so that the child can receive environmental signals in addition to the FM transmission. The problem with this or any other arrangement which incorporates the child's personal hearing aids is that when the aids break, the child is without any form of amplification. Therefore, it is usually recommended that if one of these arrangements is obtained that a set of cords and snap-on transducers, as well as snap-on earmolds, are kept for use when the aids break down.

(6) Several FM systems include a light on both the microphone/transmit-ter and the receiver which either glows or flickers when the battery is losing its charge. Younger children, in particular, frequently do not know, or will not say, when they are no longer able to hear the teacher through the FM microphone/transmitter, the environmental microphones, or both. This feature is a convenient way to visually check the battery charge during the entire day. We hate to estimate just how often children run out of sound sometime during the school day.

(7) FM auditory training systems should include a switch on the receiver unit to permit the child to receive just the teacher transmission, just the environmental signals, or both. Often, teachers will forget to turn off their microphones when the child should *not* be hearing what they are saying (sometimes to their embarrassment, as when they leave the room to talk to someone and the child is gleefully "tuned in" to a private conversation). Most FM receivers include capability for turning the teacher off (we shall have more to say about this later).

(8) At least one FM system incorporates a cardioid directional micro-phone in the teacher's transmitter. This element favors signals arriving at the teacher's microphone from her direction with a reported improvement in the signal to noise ratio arriving at the child's ear. We do not know if the theoretical advantage of this feature is superior to conventional omni-direc-tional teacher microphones under normal conditions of use (microphone 4 to 6 inches from the teacher's mouth and in the presence of an average amount of classroom noise). It is, however, a feature which does merit consideration.

(9) All FM systems include rechargeable batteries; a few, however, will also operate on a 9 volt transister radio battery. This is a useful option to have available in any emergency, such as when the charger itself is not working.

(10) A few FM systems have considered the issue of the simultaneous reception by the child of signals arriving at the teacher and the environmen-tal microphones. The specifics of how this is accomplished varies from a "muting" switch, which automatically deactivates the environmental micro-phones when the teacher is talking, a "trimmer" control, by means of which

the intensity ratio of the signals deriving from the teacher and the environmental microphones can be varied as desired, a high and constant intensity
level emanating from the teacher source and a variable child-controlled
output from the environmental microphones (but at maximum still less
intensity than from the teacher source), to evidently equal sound levels
arriving at the child's ear from both sources (given sufficiently intense environmental inputs).

At the present time, we do not know which one of these provisions would
be the most desirable under actual use conditions. The audiologist, however, should at least be aware of a how a specific FM system deals with the
problem.

(11) At least one FM instrument permits the selection of one of two
carrier wave frequencies on both the transmitter and the receiver, while
another such device allows for this option on the transmitter only. For other
systems, it is necessary to request a microphone/transmitter with a specific
carrier frequency, and 1 of 32 RO (receiver/oscillator) modules for use with
the receiver. Having the capability to instantly switch from one frequency
to another can be very useful in any school where more than one hard of
hearing child is enrolled—so is having an instantly available "loaner" microphone if necessary. The major advantage of this provision, however, would
be realized in programs where large numbers of hearing-impaired children
are enrolled; an "assembly" frequency can be common to all the children
and used for large-group communication.

(12) All FM auditory training systems make provisions for recharging the
batteries of the transmitters and the receivers. Some, however, have incorporated a few interesting extra features in the charger, such as fast and slow
recharge provisions, automatic shut-off to prevent overcharging, and troubleshooting and electroacoustic analysis circuitry. Not all of these extra
features are available in single unit chargers, however, which would likely
be the type found in schools where just one hard of hearing child is enrolled.
In instances where a larger charger is needed, such as in a resource room
for hearing-impaired children, then these extra features in the charger could
be quite useful.

Selection We view all hard of hearing children enrolled in regular
schools as potential candidates for an FM auditory training system. The
urgency of our recommendation, and the degree to which the child can
benefit depends upon the educational practices in the school and how the
school day is organized. If the school follows the classical tradition—the
teacher lecturing from up front, the children neatly lined up in rows and few
questions or discussion encouraged—an FM system can be very effective.
The hard of hearing child will be able to hear the teacher to the limits of
his auditory capacity and therefore have the same access to material as the
normally hearing children. Very few schools, to our knowledge, adhere to

this rigid kind of formalism (except perhaps colleges and universities); most display a mix of educational models including formal lectures, small group instruction centered around specific topics, and seat work or other individual activities during which the teacher circulates among the children.

The hard of hearing child can benefit from an FM transmitted speech signal during periods when the speaker's output is directed to him, whether as part of a group or individually. The FM advantage would be least during individual instruction when the teacher positions herself right next to a child, since in those circumstances the distance between the teacher and the microphone of the hearing aid would also normally be the least, thereby maximizing hearing aid reception. However, even under this condition, the teacher would not or could not position her mouth within six inches of the hearing aid microphone, which would be the distance from her mouth to the FM microphone, so the FM advantage could still be realized.

Our judgment regarding whether a child is an FM candidate depends upon the number of periods during the day the teacher's speech is directed to him, and the nature of the material covered. If the day is organized around large and small group instruction, then an FM recommendation is appropriate. We have no formulas to offer (such as, to be facetious, exposure time to the teacher's speech multiplied by the relevancy of the academic topic) to assist the teacher and clinicians in making a definitive judgment regarding a specific child's candidacy. Our experience has demonstrated that most hard of hearing children in public school settings, regardless of degree of hearing loss, will receive benefit from the proper use of an FM system. The key to success is flexibility on the part of the classroom teacher and other personnel working with the child. Our philosophy has been to look for the conditions which demonstrate the child's need for an FM system rather than vice versa. The recommendation for an FM system is usually the result of consultation among the speech-language pathologist, audiologist, and the special and classroom teacher of the hearing impaired.

Once an FM recommendation is made, then our task is to ensure that it is employed correctly. It is amazing how often these devices are used incorrectly. In the paragraphs below, we shall give a number of examples (all of which we have observed) of classroom conditions that make hearing aid usage difficult, and the appropriate and inappropriate use of an FM system in a classroom. Our intention, in presenting a large number of them, is to enable readers to deduce the general principles of correct FM auditory trainer usage in classrooms.

Difficult Classroom Conditions   Four examples are given in Figure 4–20 of typical and difficult listening conditions for a child operating in a classroom just using hearing aids. These situations were actually observed at the UConn Mainstream Project. A "traditional" situation is depicted in A; the teacher is talking, the children are generating the usual amount of classroom noise, and the child with the hearing aid (X) is receiving a speech

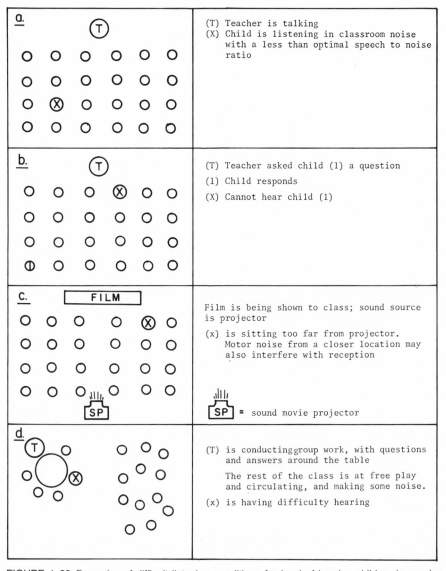

FIGURE 4–20 Examples of difficult listening conditions for hard of hearing children in regular schools when only using personal hearing aids.

to noise ratio of, at best, plus 5 dB because of the distance from the teacher and the noise in the room. In B, the situation gets a little more difficult; the teacher asks child (1) a question, and the hearing-impaired child (X) does not hear the answer, again, because of the distance and noise. In C, a film is being shown; (X) is sitting too far from the sound projector to hear; a closer location may not help that much, because of the motor noise from the projector. A written outline of the salient information would be helpful. In D, the teacher is conducting groupwork around the table with the rest of the class in free play. (X) is having difficulty hearing the questions, answers, and group discussion because of the noise the other children are making. This is a typical situation in many kindergarten rooms.

We have seen many more of these same kinds of adverse listening situations in a regular school. The acoustical and educational circumstances are normally difficult for a hard of hearing child wearing hearing aids.

Inappropriate and Appropriate Use of an FM System   In the examples portrayed in Figure 4–21, A to H, we shall give instances of incorrect use of an FM system and suggest some ways to overcome the problems given. All of these examples also have actually been observed in regular classrooms during our project.

In example A, the teacher has the FM microphone/transmitter turned on, while the child is receiving both the teacher's transmission and environmental signals (from the microphones located in the FM receiver unit worn by the child). The teacher calls on several normally hearing children to read and then asks the class a question. Another normally hearing child (1) answers the question, but very softly. The teacher says "correct" and asks the hard of hearing child for the answer, which he does not know because he has not heard it. The teacher (this is not shown in the figure) asks the normally hearing child to repeat the answer, which he does, but again very softly. The teacher says "that's right," and again asks the hard of hearing child for the answer, which again he does not know. This is not an unusual example.

We frequently observe teachers who lack insight into the listening problems experienced by a hard of hearing child. His superficially erratic behavior (sometimes he hears and responds appropriately, and sometimes he appears not to be listening or paying attention) leads many teachers to believe that the child is consciously misbehaving.

The solution in this example is simple; the teacher should have repeated the answer given by the normally hearing child. Also, if possible, and it frequently is, the FM microphone/transmitter should have been passed around to the normally hearing children who were doing the reading. Additionally, the hard of hearing child should have been seated where he can observe the other children (left or right front).

In example B, the teacher is again using the FM microphone while the child is receiving signals through both the FM and the environmental microphones. The teacher is conducting a reading group, and asks the hard of hearing child to continue reading after one of the normally hearing children (1) has finished. He is unable to do so, because he cannot hear the normally hearing child well enough to follow. This is similar in one respect to the example above; that is, the FM microphone should be passed around to the

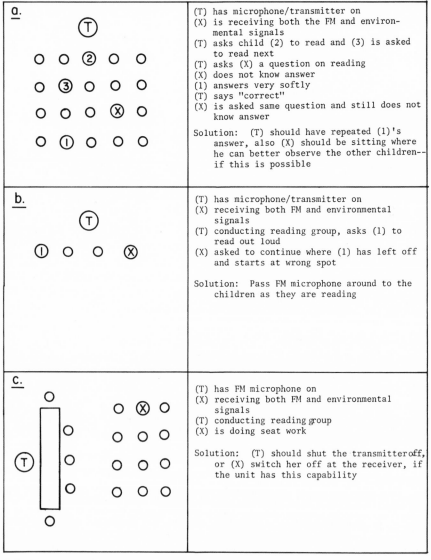

a.

(T) has microphone/transmitter on
(X) is receiving both the FM and environ-
mental signals
(T) asks child (2) to read and (3) is asked
to read next
(T) asks (X) a question on reading
(X) does not know answer
(1) answers very softly
(T) says "correct"
(X) is asked same question and still does not
know answer

Solution: (T) should have repeated (1)'s
answer, also (X) should be sitting where
he can better observe the other children--
if this is possible

b.

(T) has microphone/transmitter on
(X) receiving both FM and environmental
signals
(T) conducting reading group, asks (1) to
read out loud
(X) asked to continue where (1) has left off
and starts at wrong spot

Solution: Pass FM microphone around to the
children as they are reading

c.

(T) has FM microphone on
(X) receiving both FM and environmental
signals
(T) conducting reading group
(X) is doing seat work

Solution: (T) should shut the transmitter off,
or (X) switch her off at the receiver, if
the unit has this capability

FIGURE 4-21 Examples of incorrect use of an FM system and remediation measures.

normally hearing children as they read. It is more feasible than in the previous example because only four children are involved, and all are in close proximity to the teacher. If the classroom noise level is particularly high, it might also be advantageous to use only the teacher transmitter and when (X) is reading have him also speak into the FM microphone.

Examples C, D, E, and F are variations on the same theme. They all have in common the fact that the teacher is transmitting an FM signal during

174

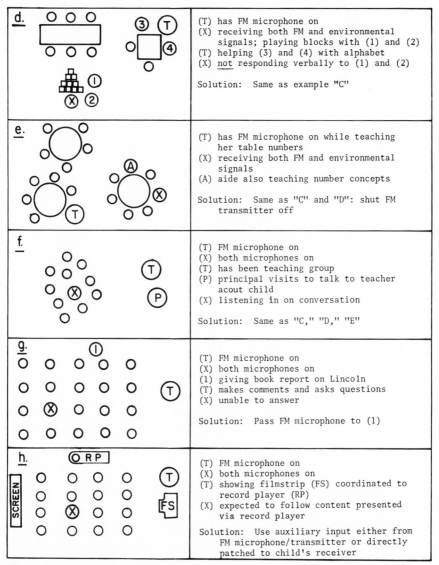

d. ⬤⬤⬤ ③ Ⓣ ⬤⬤⬤ ⬤ □ ④ ⬤ ▲ ① Ⓧ ②	(T) has FM microphone on (X) receiving both FM and environmental signals; playing blocks with (1) and (2) (T) helping (3) and (4) with alphabet (X) <u>not</u> responding verbally to (1) and (2) Solution: Same as example "C"
e.	(T) has FM microphone on while teaching her table numbers (X) receiving both FM and environmental signals (A) aide also teaching number concepts Solution: Same as "C" and "D": shut FM transmitter off
f.	(T) FM microphone on (X) both microphones on (T) has been teaching group (P) principal visits to talk to teacher acout child (X) listening in on conversation Solution: Same as "C," "D," "E"
g.	(T) FM microphone on (X) both microphones on (1) giving book report on Lincoln (T) makes comments and asks questions (X) unable to answer Solution: Pass FM microphone to (1)
h.	(T) FM microphone on (X) both microphones on (T) showing filmstrip (FS) coordinated to record player (RP) (X) expected to follow content presented via record player Solution: Use auxiliary input either from FM microphone/transmitter or directly patched to child's receiver

(Figure 4–21 continued)

periods when it is not appropriate for the hard of hearing to hear her. In one instance, C, her speech will merely be distracting; in others, D and E, her speech interferes with the child's ability to converse with other persons, and in the last such example, F, the child is listening to a private conversation. When a teacher moves some distance away from a normally hearing child, her voice intensity drops; this does not happen when the teacher is using an FM microphone. The hard of hearing child receives her speech at

175

the same intensity no matter where she is in the room. This problem—the teacher forgetting to shut the FM microphone off at certain times—is the most frequent example of inappropriate use of an FM system and the reason we have used four examples.

Example G is very similar to example B; in both the solution is to pass the microphone to the child who is doing the talking. Such a solution is not possible during rapidly alternating classroom discussions, where first one child is talking, then another, and where occasionally two or three children are talking together. Other than the child positioning himself so that he can see the faces of his classmates and being fit with the best possible electroacoustic adjustments, there is no satisfactory solution to the hearing difficulties he will experience during such conversational exchanges. Minimizing the problems ensuing from a hearing loss by correct auditory management procedures is not the same as saying we can overcome them completely.

In the last example, H, we see an instance where the auxiliary input on either the teacher's transmitter or the child's receiver should be used. Both the teacher's and the child's microphones are too far from the record player for an acceptable acoustic signal to be received. Positioning either the child, or the FM microphone closer to the record player may help a bit, but not if, as we have observed, the teacher simply places the FM microphone next to or on the record player. In this case, the unit will defect and transmit a great deal of motor noise to the child.

The major principle underlying the teacher's use of an FM system is illustrated by examples in Figure 4–21 and that is the microphone should be functioning when the teacher intends to talk to a child, as a member of a group or individually. As soon as her conversation is directed (except for occasional remarks) to other than the hard of hearing child, then the FM microphone/transmitter should be shut off. This is so simple—trivial, really—yet it is constantly violated in practice. Teachers simply forget to shut their microphone off when they should—in consequence the hard of hearing child receives inappropriate high-level speech sounds.

It is not only the teachers who should be encouraged to use the microphone, but the hard of hearing child's classmates as well. It is very often not only feasible, but positively enjoyable, for the normally hearing children to use the FM microphone when they are presenting information. It can also help to improve class discipline, since the children soon learn that "talking-time" requires the microphone. When the normally hearing children are not using the microphone, and respond to a question or make a comment, the skillful teacher will repeat what has been said (example A) for everyone's benefit, not just the hard of hearing child's.

Finally, as with the hearing aids and the FM receiver pack, the FM microphone/transmitter will do no good if it doesn't work. The teacher/clinician should charge it every night and listen to it every morning. The listening can be done quite simply by snapping the child's FM receiver into a hearing aid stethoscope or an earmold, and have a colleague talk through the FM microphone from across the room. It would be an instructive experience to ask the colleague to gently bump the unit onto her desk or the blackboard, as would normally occur when a teacher is working at her desk or at the blackboard, and listen for the resulting noise explosions. Such an experience can help the teachers realize the sensitivity of the FM microphone/transmitter to vibrations and excessive physical handling.

section summary

In summary, we have presented in this section a model of audiological management of hard of hearing children in schools. We consider this topic the therapeutic "front-line" in their overall management, to be reinforced and supported by any other therapeutic measure necessary to achieve our ultimate objective—a child who is fulfilling his intellectual and psychosocial potential in spite of his handicap. The foundation having been laid, we can now turn to these other therapeutic considerations.

○ SPEECH AND LANGUAGE MANAGEMENT

In the previous section, we stressed the need to capitalize fully on the child's residual hearing. Therapeutic intervention in the speech and language areas should, however, proceed simultaneously with auditory management because those latter efforts are a never-ending focus throughout the child's school career.

The specific goals we select for therapeutic intervention obviously relate to the results of the comprehensive performance evaluation. Those problems which interfere most with a child's communication efforts are usually attacked first, but not always. Sometimes it makes sense to initially concentrate on difficulties which can be remediated relatively easily; success with these problems can provide the needed level of motivation for the child (and the therapist) in the more intensive exertions required to solve more difficult problems. Specific therapy goals, moreover, should reflect a developmental, child-oriented view of speech and language, rather than an adult, finished-product orientation. The evidence is clear that speech and language development accompanies perceptual and cognitive maturation; it would therefore be unwise to impose linguistic demands upon a child before he is ready for them.

The child, in other words, must first have something to say—that is, he must be able to cognitively appreciate his experiences before we concern ourselves with the specific language forms he uses to code these experiences. Indeed, the linguistic deficiencies displayed by many a hard of hearing child can be conceptualized as having their base in an impoverished quality and quantity of relevant experiences, rather than being the inevitable outcome of the hearing loss itself. The response to the child's hearing loss becomes the occasion for reducing, consciously or unconsciously, the richness of the child's life experiences instead of the opposite. These children need more, not less. Accompanying, therefore, the specific linguistic goals we select to begin therapy is an awareness of the motivating and meaningful experiences we can create and utilize—experiences to which the language forms are associated. Language has a purpose; we are not apt to be very successful clinicians if we divorce the forms we attempt to teach a child from the nonlinguistic content the forms encode in a communicative situation.

In working with a hard of hearing child, we have advantages not usually evident with normally hearing children who display speech and language deviations. First, in distinction to many of these other children, we have a clear-cut understanding of the reason for the hard of hearing child's problems (excluding multiply handicapped children, for whom the situation may not be quite so clear). How often, in working with normally hearing children who show communication problems, can we ascribe the child's difficulties to a specific etiological condition? Knowing the precise reason for a child's problems certainly makes the planning of a therapeutic program a more rational affair.

Secondly, again in contradistinction to these other children, we can assume that the hard of hearing child possesses a normal central perceptual and cognitive capacity for learning speech and language. Faced with a child whose communication problems arise because of a central disorganization or defect, we would find it very difficult to know where to begin or how to proceed; with the hard of hearing child, on the other hand, whose biological capacity for learning speech and language is presumably intact (particularly for the younger child who should display more neurological plasticity), we can employ this capacity as our greatest natural therapy ally.

Our task, as we have reviewed earlier, is to minimize the impact of the peripheral hearing loss upon the child's innate abilities. Given this accomplishment, our therapeutic objectives can often be met simply by arranging a rich and repeated exposure to the proper experiences (acoustic/phonetic, nonlinguistic, and linguistic), and correcting only when such a naturalistic approach is already too late, unsuccessful, or must be fine tuned.

In the following pages, we shall discuss the management of five general areas in which the hard of hearing child often displays problems. These areas are vocabulary, syntax, language usage, speech reception, and speech production intelligibility. In practice, it is very difficult to isolate one area of concern from another; just as they are all interwoven in the child's utterances, so in remediation it may be difficult to isolate problems which cut across more than one area.

Good therapy practice, however, dictates that focus be placed at any given time on only one clearly defined therapy goal. Children must know what is expected of them. For example, while trying to arrange experiences to foster the induction of some complex syntactic structure, it is advisable to use only familiar lexical items in the sentence. The corollary is also applicable; while teaching new vocabulary in a sentence frame, it is advisable to employ only known syntactic constructions. There is no significance therefore to the order in which we have chosen to discuss the five general areas. This applies even to the traditional precedence given speech perception ("ear") training to speech production therapy; with the hard of hearing child, these two areas are also so interwoven that in reality a great deal of alternating emphases take place.

teaching vocabulary

Most hard hearing children manifest some limitations in their vocabulary development; many of them demonstrate quite severe problems. For normally hearing children, vocabulary growth proceeds almost as effortlessly as does grammatical development. While their caretakers often label objects and occurrences in the child's environment, as a part of the normal child–caretaker linguistic interaction, many new lexical items, as well as the reinforcement of words they have already been exposed to, are learned through the continued auditory exposure to language. A normally hearing child can be "tuned in" to language spoken anywhere in his auditory field; all parents know how often children hear and employ words they are not supposed to know and use! Much of this vocabulary development (and, of course, linguistic development in general) proceeds unconsciously, as a kind of auditory osmosis associated with the pertinent nonlinguistic experiences. It is important to realize that vocabulary growth normally continues throughout the life of an individual; not so with syntactic development, which shows few changes (particularly in oral communication) after the elementary years.

For the hard of hearing child, on the other hand, a restricted lexicon may very well be more injurious to his ultimate ability to communicate effectively than his grammatical deficiencies—unless these are particularly severe. He will not usually learn a new word unless it is specifically directed to him in the proper kind of motivating and acoustic circumstances. When a group of normally hearing children crowd around an ice cream truck, asking for all kinds of exotic flavors, the hard of hearing child cannot hear, discriminate, or associate their requests with a specific flavor, so he may just restrict his choice to vanilla (the white ice cream) or chocolate (the brown kind).

Examples such as this one can be extended at length; it is surprising, and somewhat distressing, to learn how many common words hard of hearing children do not know. We know of one youngster who used the words "Kool

Aid," sometimes modified by a color adjective, to request all types of beverages other than milk, simply because he did not know, and was not taught at expeditious times, the proper labels for other types of beverages.

It is rare for hard of hearing children to read any kind of book for the sheer pleasure of it, simply because their comprehension is poor. One can even recommend an intense regime of comic books for many hard of hearing children, not because the content is approved, but because the pictures aid in the comprehension of the printed word and the children can thereby develop positive associations with reading. Eventually, reading is apt to be their greatest entree into the linguistic world and such positive associations can be of inestimable value.

Normally hearing children can ordinarily figure out, even though sometimes with difficulty, the meaning of new words from the linguistic context; not so many hard of hearing children, for whom the context (lexical and grammatical) may be as unfamiliar as the new word. School children are exposed to new vocabulary at an awesome rate in such areas as reading, social studies, and science; getting the meaning of a new word, retaining it, and processing it automatically is a difficult task under the best of circumstances. The meager linguistic resources of many hard of hearing children do not permit them to effectively employ the linguistic context to gain comprehension of the new words they meet in school. This situation seems to get worse beginning at about the fourth or fifth grade; beyond this, a hard of hearing child may fall further and further behind unless he receives an intensive individualized tutorial program. The child's vocabulary deficiencies, moreover, are not limited to school-based words. It also reflects gaps in knowledge of common everyday words—those expected of a child when he enters school.

In our view, this problem occurs primarily because of exposure limitations. In order to facilitate the communication process, normally hearing children and adults often modify their linguistic input to hard of hearing children, and thus restrict or distort the crucial linguistic exposures necessary for the development of both oral and written vocabulary. Parents, in particular, often continue to use a simplified lexicon with their children since they can thereby be assured of transmitting their message accurately. While the intent is positive, the results may very well be negative in terms of their child's vocabulary growth.

General Principles In attempting to expand the functional vocabulary of a hard of hearing child, a number of general principles apply and must be considered. As explained above, our general philosophy of speech and language management is basically a developmental one in a naturalistic framework. To be most effective, we must permit the child's cognitive and maturation levels, interests, needs, and motivations, to guide us both in the procedures we adopt and the specific vocabulary items we select for therapy. Beyond this, society (through the medium of the child's school and out of school environment) has evolved expectations of vocabulary performance which must also guide us in the selection of specific therapy goals. These considerations offer us a range of therapeutic possibilities. Within them, the astute clinician can find those words which are most necessary for a child and will therefore make the greatest difference in his performance, as well as recognize those words that can best serve the child's own perceived needs and interests and, which, therefore, engage his motivated learning.

In learning any new word, a great deal of repetition, redundancy, rephrasing and a host of varied associations are necessary. We cannot expect a child to fully comprehend and employ new words after only one or two exposures. They have to be presented repeatedly in many different contexts, such as matching words to definitions, crossword puzzles, verbal riddles, and through the intensive use of a word dictionary or thesaurus.

When possible, vocabulary items should be taught with objects or actions which require the active participation of the child. For example, in learning words which code the concepts of possession, action, location, or time—for which he probably already possesses the cognitive readiness—it is possible to employ physical objects (putting things "in" or "on" something, or "there" or "here," taking an action "before" or "later") and real experiences ("building," "cutting," "tearing," "pasting") to convey the concept to a child. At a later stage, when more abstract words are learned ("assistance") it is true, words may have to be used to define other words, but even at this point, situations and examples that give a context can be contrived to illustrate the meaning of a word.

For the hard of hearing child, it is imperative that new words be presented both auditorially and in printed form (preferably in that order), and that the child can make the necessary associations. This is particularly important when the form of the written word does not reflect standard pronunciation and it is learned first. In these instances, confusion can arise when the child hears the word in its spoken form (doubt, ghost, thought, rough). This error occurs frequently in spelling exercises.

We would like to reach the point where the child's linguistic development is sufficient for him to use the printed word as a major avenue for vocabulary (and, less so, syntactic) development. We do not expect a child to recite the definition of a new word upon request; normally hearing children cannot accomplish this task very well either. Repetition and review must permeate every lesson, even more than we would expect to do with a normally hearing child, simply because the hard of hearing child's subsequent auditory exposure to the new words is apt to be minimal. Our goal is to reach the point where the child can automatically and unconsciously comprehend and employ the new vocabulary items, both in oral and written forms.

Approaches to Word Selection (1) The speech-language pathologist should consult with all the child's teachers and secure from them a list
of words which all the children in the class are expected to know. These can
relate to past lessons or activities, or simply be words specific to the school
situation (for example such words as "recess," "erase," "monitor," "discipline," "vice-principal," "secretary" and so on). One cannot assume that
the hard of hearing child understands the use of words which are specific
to the school situation unless he can explicitly demonstrate it. In addition,
the teachers should be queried regarding observations they have made of
words that the child seemed not to understand. All special teachers should
be asked to compile a vocabulary list specific to their specialty, such as
"easel," "canvas," and "kiln" for the art teacher, the names of the different
instruments and musical terms for the music teacher, and "stacks," "ency-
clopedia," and "directory" for the librarian. These words deal with expectations—this is the lexicon mastered by his hearing classmates, which he must
also comprehend and use.

The speech-language pathologist then determines whether the hard of
hearing child understands and can use the word. We suggest that this be
accomplished by having the child use it in a sentence, or through an appropriate action ("pouring," "mixing," or "stirring" something, or miming
being "furious," "joyful," or "fatigued"). This determination must be made
for any vocabulary item selected by the above step or by any of the other
procedures enumerated below. For example, after a chapter on light, the
following words were selected for emphasis. The child was asked to use
these words in a fill in the blank exercise:

photons	concave	spectrum
opaque	convex	prism
transparent	mirage	lenses
translucent	refraction	retina

(2) The child is asked to read material taken from the curriculum which
he has, or shortly will, be exposed to and to underline any word that he does
not fully comprehend. The speech-language pathologist goes through the
same material and underlines those additional words the child may have
difficulty with. Subject areas such as social studies and science, which cover
a lot of vocabulary in a short time, should be prime targets for this approach.
It is a good practice to include some words which the child does understand,
to give him some experiences of success when he is asked to define them
(again, through actions or in a sentence). These children know they have
problems; once in a while some positive reinforcement, even if it has to be
contrived, can boost their self-image and improve their motivation.

(3) The speech-language pathologist should extract the vocabulary dealing with the language of directions from the child's seat-work lessons, workbooks and both standardized and local tests. We have already discussed the difficulty many of these children have with this task. Often, this language is more complex than the tasks themselves and their subsequent failure may relate more to difficulty in comprehending the directions rather than the tasks themselves. Such words and phrases as "underline," "circle," "match," "connect," "fill-in," "complete" may be inadequately comprehended by a child.

A test such as the Boehm Test of Basic Concepts includes direction vocabulary which has been empirically validated on normally hearing children of different ages (at the kindergarten, first and second grade for the Boehm test). Such tests do not *sample* the child's performance, as the PPVT does, but rather establish certain *standards* of knowledge which the child must meet. As such, they can serve as a criterion-referenced task to direct the teaching goals of the speech-language pathologist.

Below is listed the direction vocabulary from two reading workbooks which can serve as vocabulary goals:

study	pattern	rewrite	work up or down	add
trace	sentence	in order	that fit	grow
copy	finish	tell	story	another
compare	scrambled	missing	work across	

underline	phrase	opposite	set	large
belong	blank	space	right	alike
group	fill	spell	check	
correct	make a list	correctly	first	
doesn't belong	think	appropriate	column	
complete	rhymes	below	small	

As an example of typical instructions, consider the following:
The *pronouns* in the following *passage* are *underlined* and *numbered.* Write the *word* or *phrase* that each pronoun *stands for after* the *corresponding* number *below* the *passage.* *

After each *incomplete sentence below,* there is a *pronoun* in *parentheses.* To make that pronoun *fit in* the *sentence blank,* you may have to change the *form* of it.**

(4) The most motivating vocabulary to select in working with a hard of hearing child is that he selects himself. By this we do not mean that the child brings a list of words to the clinician which he wants explained, but rather

---

*SRA Reading Program—Level L
**A. Schiller et al., *Language and How To Use It,* Glenview, Ill.: Scott, Foresman, and Co.

where the child is asked to discuss his interests, activities, and hobbies with the speech-language pathologist. If the child enjoys putting airplane or automobile models together, he has probably been depending mostly upon the pictured rather than the written directions (and making many errors). The clinician and child can jointly work on the task, with the child reading and attempting to follow the written directions while being assisted by the clinician (assuming that the clinician knows how to put models together!). If the child collects rocks, coins, stamps, or bottle tops; if he is interested in natural history and possibly keeps a few gerbils at home or has an aquarium; if the antics of the latest group of rock stars, or the newest hit on TV fascinates him; whatever his interests or whatever turns him on (within limits) can be grist for the vocabulary mill.

In using a child's self-selected interests as a mechanism for vocabulary management, however, it is important that the speech-language pathologist not turn the child's communication efforts off with constant corrections— particularly for the younger hard of hearing child. In teaching vocabulary, our goal is to foster communication, not to impede it. For the younger child, the needed and new vocabulary can be modeled repeatedly by the clinician —in many variations and concrete circumstances—as the primary teaching device.

The child taking driver's education might select the following vocabulary:

Parts of car	Action words
steering wheel	speeding
gear shift	overheat
speedometer	shifting
windshield wipers	steering
seat belts	backing up
clutch	forward
brake	reverse
engine	fill up
battery	check under the hood
radiator	check oil
blinker	tune-up
	parallel park
	back up
	park

(5) All children want to play games, in and out of school; many, emulating their parents and peers, are avid sports followers. The vocabulary associated with the rules of the games, the accomplishments of various teams and players, offer a unique opportunity to capture the interest of a child in a vocabulary management program. In a football game, for example, the child may know the reasons for certain events, but not know the associated verbal labels; such words as "foul," "penalty," "offside," "huddle," "block," "in-

tercept," "goal posts," "end" to define a playing position or, "end-run," "half-time," "quarter time," and so on.

Each game has its special vocabulary, and if a child is to discuss or follow a game intelligently, or if he is to meet his peers on a relatively equal basis, he must know the definitions of these words. A more immediate need for the average hard of hearing child is to ensure that he understands the rules of the games played in the school yard and in his neighborhood. We have known hard of hearing children who avoided, or were excluded from, games simply because they did not know the rules.

Hearing children absorb such rules relatively easily; they can hear or already know the special lexicon and the verbal explanation. The hard of hearing child may know the concept of a "sacrifice" (in a baseball game) or a "bunt." He may even hear his "coach" (one of the other children) tell him to make those plays. He just may not have met these words, and others, often enough to understand them, and therefore he makes the wrong moves to the disgust of his teammates. Teaching such a child the meaning of the special vocabulary associated with the games he participates in, or would like to if he could, may transcend the undisputed importance of learning academic material. The child's self-image and social adjustment is tied to his ability to participate in games with his hearing peers on equal terms. This vocabulary is needed to fully participate in baseball including understanding the rules:

home	outfield	tag
home base	right field	slide
1st	center field	bunt
1st base	left field	pop up
2nd base	foul line	out
3rd base	pitcher	strike
basemen	catcher	ball
play 1st (2nd,	back stop	homerun
3rd) base	pop fly	homer
shortstop	fly	safe

(6) For the less active clinician, or the one who could never quite grasp the intrinsic fascination that hitting, kicking, or throwing a ball around has for most of our society, the use of board games within the confines of the therapy room can be an effective device for vocabulary enhancement (but not really a substitute for most children). This is an old and time-honored therapy standby, but nonetheless potentially valuable when employed by a clinician who knows how to use the activity to assess and remediate a child's vocabulary deficiencies. Indeed, many board games are specifically designed with vocabulary enhancement in mind. It is a good idea, however, to verify with other kinds of activities any new words arising out of a picture-based

board game. This is to ensure that the child's understanding of such words are not restricted to the particular context in which they were learned.

The variety of board games currently available enable the clinician to concentrate on many different facets of a child's difficulties. Some include sorting words according to categories, such as occupations, transportation, food, and appliances; others employ problem solving activities, make use of verbal analogies and reasoning, and require inferential reasoning. It is also possible to devise simple board games using whatever category of lexical items are pertinent—for example, money names (penny, nickel, dime), sports events (tennis, javelin).

Properly used, they permit the speech-language pathologist to supply useful vocabulary to a child in a moderately relevant context during periods of high motivation (what child does not enjoy being pulled out of class to play games!). For each new lexical item, the clinician should expose the child to both the oral and written forms, and then verify his comprehension by employing it and eliciting its use in other contexts.

Vocabulary needed for a board game:

spin	win	dice
spinner	roll	go to jail
turn	jump own man	go past go
man	king	pay the bank
forward	move	deed
back	shuffle	hotel
lose	card	

(7) In every activity with a child, conversation should be taking place. During such exchanges with a child, the speech-language therapist should note what words were used incorrectly or with an unintended nuance and at what point the child had word-finding problems and perhaps circumlocuted or used an inordinate amount of pronouns. Ordinarily, one would think that if a child used such forms as demonstrative or indefinite pronouns, that this would suggest a sophisticated mastery of the language. For hard of hearing children, however, this may not be true. They tend to use such words as "that," "this," "these," "those," "it," when they are unable to label the proper reference because of their vocabulary limitations. This usage is frequently accepted by their parents or peers as long as the intended information is conveyed. It should not be accepted by the speech-language pathologist who should determine if the child knows the label for the pronoun referent.

Offering the child the proper label (though not necessarily requiring the child to imitate it) when they use an indefinite or demonstrative pronoun or when they employ such strategies as "you know" or "thing," supplies him with the word he needs at a psychologically appropriate time. It is then appropriate to set up a situation in which the child is obliged to use the new item presented. Motivation is maximum, and the new word can be spoken immediately in a relevent communicative situation.

(8) *The Basic Vocabulary and Language Thesaurus* developed by Ling and Ling (1977), which contains more than 2000 words listed according to their frequency of usage by normally hearing children, can be employed to provide goals in a vocabulary management program. The hard of hearing children should be expected to comprehend and use all the words in this thesaurus.

Other word categories which can serve as training material are lists of antonyms and synonyms. From a semantic point of view, it is difficult for a child to truly understand a word unless he can also comprehend its opposite (try explaining the meaning of the word "rough" without also covering "smooth"!). A number of lists of antonyms and synonyms are commercially available. A vocabulary list of synonyms can logically lead to lessons concerning multiple meanings of individual words. This is something that many hard of hearing children have difficulty with. They are often able to employ a word in a very narrow or specific sense yet not know that the same word, in a different or even a similar kind of linguistic context, can embody other meanings as well (the word "hot," for example, can refer to heat, anger, excitement, proximity, a stolen item, zealousness, or lust; any child or person, who can employ this word only to convey the concept of excessive temperature has cut himself off from a great deal of human communication). Finally, words referring to a category of things or events are useful inclusions in a vocabulary training program (for example, in transportation, food, clothing, and occupations).

(9) Hard of hearing children need a great deal of exposure and practice with idiomatic expressions if they are to be "with it" in conversation with their peers. As with metaphorical expressions, one cannot literally decode the individual words to arrive at the intended meaning, but must learn them through structured exposure in context. Phrases like, "under the weather," "frog in your throat," "chip on your shoulder," "pain in the neck" require such a context. Slang such as "you turkey" or "gross" are not apt to be used by the adults in their world, and in their peer contacts the expressions may not have been heard often enough, or clearly enough, to be understood.

Words with multiple, frequently nonliteral, meanings also give them a great deal of difficulty ("run" is a good example of such a word). The situations which require the use of the different meanings in the varied context in which they are employed have to be experienced by the children as much as possible ("running" for president or a "running" nose). Normally hearing elementary aged school children have an obsession (or so it seems to us) for the riddles and jokes (Question: Why is a room full of married people like an empty room? Answer: Because there is not a single person in it). While this kind of riddle or joke can drive adults crazy, kids love it, and it can expand their language horizons. Riddle or joke books are available in most bookstores. A typical feature of such books is the verbal absurdity component of the jokes and riddles, which is another area hard of hearing children have problems with. The use of such books in therapy is a very motivating, and as much as we hate to say it, a relevant teaching tool—provided, of course, the child knows when and to whom it would be appropriate to tell the jokes and riddles.

In short, arriving at specific goals for increasing the vocabulary knowledge of hard of hearing children is a relatively simple task. As outlined above, the speech-language pathologist can employ many assessment and remediation procedures. The more difficult task is to establish priorities, and in this it is not possible to recommend a specific sequence of vocabulary goals. Each hard of hearing child will demonstrate different capabilities and gaps. We can be most effective with a motivated child; and therefore the child's interests and needs must be explored. Beyond this, however, we have to focus on the vocabulary items which can make the greatest difference in the child's performance, that is those words which his world (school and home) expects him to know.

syntax management

Unlike that of "deaf" children, the spoken syntax used by hard of hearing children often appears to be superficially adequate (with individual exceptions, of course). In a face-to-face conversational situation, the hard of hearing child has the option of selecting from a number of potentially suitable linguistic structures and strategies for communication purposes. To assist in accurate comprehension of the message, the child can utilize the normal redundancy in spoken utterance as well as a number of nonlinguistic cues. Any syntactic problems, therefore, that the child demonstrates do not appear to seriously disrupt the oral communication process.

Syntactic problems, however, will become evident in the child's school work as he progresses through the elementary grades because his reading and writing skills will reflect his auditory-based language development. This justifies our concern with the syntactic level of a young hard of hearing child, even with those children for whom the syntactic deviations and simplifications do not seriously interfere with their oral communication. It is also more efficient to attempt to place a child on the right syntactic development path when they are young, when their aptitude for such a development is at its peak. For older children, and for those whose syntactic competency is clearly deficient, our therapeutic intervention requires no such justification. Our experience is that hard of hearing children do not self-correct habituated syntactic errors unless they are helped.

There is a clear relationship between the syntactic problems of hard of hearing children and the configuration and extent of a hearing loss. It is important to distinguish between those children who do not know the meaning of the morphological ending and those who know the meaning but omit the endings for acoustic reasons. The following example shows how the same behavior can be produced for different reasons, which leads to different management techniques:

BEHAVIOR	REASON	MANAGEMENT SUGGESTIONS
no use of plural /s/ "I saw two cat"	does not know plural rule (linguistic)	teach plural rule by example
no use of plural /s/ "I saw two cat"	knows plural rule but consistently omits final /s/ because it is hard to hear (acoustic)	practice discriminating plural vs. nonplural practice monitoring own production of plural vs. nonplural

Morphological endings are ordinarily unstressed in a conversational utterance—that is, they are weaker in intensity than the words to which they are attached (for example, the past tense /ed/). The child has difficulty in detecting the acoustic correlate of the suffix and therefore cannot easily learn its meaning. In addition, many function words, verb forms, and contractions are similarly unstressed in speech. In such utterances as, "where's he going," "he's walked home," "let's go in there," "he's got the boat," "he's got a boat," "he's got some boats," "the teacher's in the room" or "the teacher's room," the hard of hearing child will find it difficult to hear the contracted and assimilated forms of the verbs, articles, and function words.

An additional complication for many hard of hearing children is the high frequency composition of many of these elements, which make them much more difficult to detect. Thus the hard of hearing child will have difficulty inducing the correct grammatical rules from conversational samples and learning to employ them appropriately. Some of these elements are also very difficult to speechread (for example, the article "a," the preposition "in," and the /s/ and the /t/ endings, particularly in a high front vowel environment where the lip opening is minimal).

We are once again emphasizing the genesis of these children's language problems because the main course of our therapeutic approach follows directly from our understanding of the etiology. Not only do these children have difficulty in detecting specific linguistic elements, but they are in general *exposed* to a reduced complexity and quantity of relevant language input. The people in their environment commonly tend to talk down to them, to emphasize what the children can easily understand. The child achieves a level of communicative competence with which he can get by as he talks to peers, teachers, and parents who can understand him. Because he communicates, we tend to accept the child's level of communication performance. We thus reduce his exposure to new forms and encourage him to remain at a lower level of syntactic performance.

A prime example of this exposure concept can be observed in the difficulty hard of hearing children have in learning passive constructions. We generally converse in the active and not the passive voice, because of English conversational constraints, so the hard of hearing child does not receive sufficient exposure to the passive form to become fluent in its use. Perhaps if we talked in a passive and not an active sense ("the boy was bitten by the dog," rather than "the dog bit the boy") it would be the active construction which would give hard of hearing children difficulty. The main focus of our therapeutic approach, therefore, can be conveyed in the one word *"exposure."*

We are not recommending a regime of just talk, talk, talk. While we emphasize discourse as the key factor in syntax therapy, we are not suggesting that the child simply be bombarded with conversation, that his world view be limited to moving lips and a monotonous drone. For the child to induce the linguistic rules of the language, the enriched exposure he receives must be relevant to the nonlinguistic events that he is experiencing and that concern him. Furthermore, such exposure must occur when he is developmentally ready and motivated to receive it. It is not a good idea to attempt to teach a syntactic rule by explaining it verbally to a child. Certainly, after a while the child can be taught to recite the rule, but unless he has worked out for himself the relationships between the nonlinguistic and linguistic events—or he knows what it is he wants to communicate and the necessary linguistic forms to achieve this purpose—the generalization or carry-over to nontherapeutic situations will be minimal.

The following example shows how an adult can expose the child to the correct linguistic forms during the course of an ordinary conversation.

Modelling example:

Child: "Where going?"	*Adult*: Where *is* she going?
C: Yeh.	*A*: She'*s* going to get some soda. Where *is* he going?
C: He going outside.	*A*: Oh, he *is going* outside. *I'm going* outside too. Where *are* you going?
C: I'm going outside too.	*A*: Let's go!

If the speech-language pathologist understands the child's linguistic deficiencies and understands that they, for the hard of hearing child, are not normally based on deviations in cognitive development, it should not be too difficult to arrange experiences to facilitate his induction on specific linguistic rules. For example, if a child has difficulty in comprehending or employing one sentence embedded into another (complementation or relativization), situations can be contrived which require him to select "the boy who was chasing the dog fell down" from an array of pictures showing a boy chasing a dog which falls, a dog chasing a boy who falls, and a boy and a dog both falling. After experiencing a number of these tasks and responding correctly, he can be asked to generate similar sentences when exposed to similar experiences (through models, actions on his part, or pictures). Other situations can be contrived which require him to respond to any linguistic structure he has problems with, such as possession, the proper use of articles, tense, contractions, and the third person /s/. The life situation of a child or the common therapy materials available should afford the creative clinician ample opportunities to contrive relevant experiences.

In order for a child to learn any syntactic construction causing difficulty, he requires *repeated* exposures to the construction in a meaningful situation. In the early stages of therapy, the clinician has to increase the saliency of the input, by exaggerating the stress, intonation or duration with which she expresses the specific linguistic construction. The rate of input can be slowed to give the child a better opportunity to process the presence of the elements he has difficulty perceiving. Later, as the child is learning that "something" is there which conveys a necessary meaning, a more normal mode of input can be assumed. When the child reaches the point that he can recognize the correct form in other's speech, he should be exposed to occasional incorrect versions and asked to judge when a form is or is not correct, and if not, to correct it. Our goal here is to encourage the monitoring of spoken messages, of others and himself. A great deal of exposure is required before a child can reach this point, but once it is done, the linguistic rule has been automotized by the child and we can go on to other problems.

In the course of these repeated exposures, many hard of hearing children begin to develop functional knowledge of linguistic rules we have not explicitly taught them. This is a heartening development, since it shows that the child has begun to expand his auditory processing beyond the limits of the specific forms we have been concentrating on. Attempting to isolate and explicitly teach the myriad of linguistic forms a child may have problems with can be a hopeless frustrating endeavor. We must engage the child's innate capacities for inducing the rules of the language. There is no better way to do this than ensuring the repeated, rephrased, auditory, exposures occur in meaningful situations.

Once the child begins to gain understanding of a rule, written representations should be employed, not before. The child is asked to read and select the appropriate construction from a number of incorrect ones; similarly, he is required to write the correct form after being exposed to the eliciting situations. Reading is a marvelous avenue for the hard of hearing child to expand his language as well as his intellectual vistas. Before they can approach reading for this purpose, however, they must possess a sufficient level of competency to enable the known context to clarify the meaning of unknown or unclear structures. Additionally, the type of language a child will meet in reading is not the same as he uses, or is expected to use, in oral communication. For both these reasons, it is advisable to initially stress auditory language development and then base written lessons on the progress of this development. When it appears that a child can use the context of a reading lesson to deduce the meaning and usage of unknown forms (as well as new vocabulary), then reading assignments can play a major role in syntax therapy. We would like to see such a child read just for the fun of it.

facilitating language usage

The hard of hearing child must be able to employ language for communication purposes. Learning to use a language means being able to make inferences about the differences in social and contextual situations and then code these differences with unique linguistic forms. Knowing a language code is relevant only if the child can employ it in varying contexts for different purposes. Ordinarily, we expect a child to learn the proper use of a linguistic form concurrently with his associations with relevant experience. Such expectations do not hold for hard of hearing children. Their exposures to linguistic forms are insufficiently audible, diversified, or frequent to permit them to unconsciously induce the rules of language usage. The hard of hearing child will know when he intends to request an action, information, permission, or help; he understands the differences between a warning, a threat, an invitation, or a promise; he may not, however, be able to select the proper linguistic form to express these intentions, or know how to modify the expressions in different situations for listeners who possess different degrees of prior knowledge.

Many hard of hearing chidren are unable to react sensitively and selectively to the feedback given them by listeners. Most hard of hearing children simply repeat an identical sentence, perhaps just saying it louder when a listener implicitly or explicitly indicates that the message was incompletely or incorrectly understood. They must be taught how to paraphrase and to be sensitive to a listener's needs during a two-way conversation.

Much progress in this dimension of language will be a by-product of the enriched linguistic exposures in relevant experiential frameworks, which we have already discussed in vocabulary and syntax management. The social contexts in which these therapies take place define the language usage dimension. We cannot, however, expect a child to efficiently learn language usage rules only as a by-product of our other therapeutic efforts. Some manipulation of the situation is necessary in order to focus on specific usage problems as well as to provide the intensive practice required for automatizing the rules.

An effective procedure for enhancing and facilitating language usage is to arrange role playing activities, with the clinician periodically interchanging roles with the child so as to generate correct usage models for the child. Dolls, pictures, or just imagination can be employed under a large variety of situations. Scenarios can be contrived in which:

(1) The child assumes different roles in giving direction, information, or asking questions. This activity will demonstrate that people employ different linguistic constructions in talking to different people under different circumstances.

(2) The clinician assumes two roles, perhaps a teacher and a child, with the child required to interpose comments at the proper time, expand or add information to an utterance, and make inferences from the communication exchange. For example, the clinician may assume the role of a child asking a teacher why he received such a poor grade, with the teacher responding, "you know very well" (did not do his homework, behaved poorly, copied on a test). In other situations, the child can be asked "what is that man thinking," or "why did he do that?", or "what happens next." Making inferences from given information is often difficult for hard of hearing children, particularly from reading, and this kind of activity can help them develop their inferential abilities.

(3) Different kinds of given and known information are contrived. The child is expected to modify his language usage to reflect what both speakers know and do not know in some situation. For example, the "mother" says that the ice cream is in the freezer and the child has to request that "it" be taken out, or when "a," "the," "this," "that," or "some" is used to modify the word "boy" in some situation, and the child has to select the right stimulus picture.

(4) The differences between such concepts as "ask" and "tell," and "bring" and "take" can be conveyed. For example, in a mock party, a child can "tell" his younger brother that he can not come, but "ask" or "invite" his friends; "promise" his mother that he will behave; "warn" his kid brother that he had better behave ("after" his mother "made" him be included), "wonder" what kind of presents the children will "bring," and "buy" party favors for them to "take" home.

(5) The child has to understand that there are different ways of expressing the same intention under different circumstances. In the role the clinician plays, she can say to her "mother," "I wish I had some ice cream," "is there any ice cream?", "I want ice cream," "give me some," "that looks good," and work out with the child the situations in which the different usages would be correct (i.e., has the best chance of getting the desired

object). In the course of this kind of activity, the differences between direct, indirect, and inferred requests can be demonstrated as well as the circumstances in which each is appropriate.

(6) The child is asked to describe the same activity a number of different ways. This is very important because the hard of hearing child will frequently meet with different verbal expressions conveying the same information; he also must frequently rephrase his utterances when people do not understand him. He can, for example, imagine explaining the same game to a blind child, one who sees, one who is already somewhat familiar with the game, a much younger child, a stranger, a foreigner. A situation can be contrived in which a communication failure has occurred (the "listener" taking the wrong action or responding inappropriately). The child must then practice saying the same message in different ways; this gives him practice in strategies for handling listener-feedback responses.

(7) The older hard of hearing child, who requires a more sophisticated grasp of the rules of language usage, can be asked to "imagine" how he would ask the new girl on the block for a date, or how to respond when someone asks him or her to go to the junior prom. Current events can be brought into the role playing situation with the older child, who is asked to assume the roles of different figures in the news.

(8) A communication game can be developed to teach the child the necessity of presenting clear, and specifically adapted, messages to a listener. A dyad (speaker and listener) is seated at opposite sides of a table divided by a small screen which allows for eye contact between the two participants. Traditionally (Flavell 1975), the speaker and listener are given the same set of nonsense figures which are placed so that the listener cannot see the speaker's choice. It then becomes the speaker's responsibility to describe the chosen nonsense figure with sufficient exactitude to permit the listener to select the corresponding item. If the message is not sufficiently precise, or not adapted to the listener's perspective, then the communication attempt has failed and must be revised for success.

The above format can be adapted in a variety of ways to use as a vehicle for improving communication skills in hearing-impaired children. It is possible to devise a situation in which the speaker has a visual pattern in front of him that he must describe in sufficient and accurate detail to enable a listener to graphically replicate the pattern. As long as the speaker is allowed to see the listener's response, feedback regarding the accuracy of his description is immediately available. The child's awareness of imprecise message transmission (negative feedback), as well as the strategy he used to revise his message, can be analyzed and remedied using this procedure. It is interesting to note that many hard of hearing children blame the listener for the communication failure rather than their own inaccurate message. The use of previously drawn maps indicating specific paths to be taken to reach a goal is another variation which allows for analysis regarding the child's sensitivity to a listener response and the kind of strategy used to modify messages and ensure comprehension.

(9) Because of the difficulty that many hearing-impaired children have in learning socially appropriate conversational skills, it is desirable to demonstrate correct procedures for entering a conversation, changing topics, interrupting, and turn taking. Some of these children have learned an adult initiated question/answer routine that limits any response on their part to a single sentence. It may be necessary to help a child redesign a previous conversation to make him realize the accuracy and advantages of a discourse conversational format. Practice in just carrying on extended conversations should increase a childs communicative competence and promote their acceptance into a mainstream setting.

Above all, to learn to use language for communication purposes, the hard of hearing child must be exposed to a great variety of it, in a warm interpersonal setting (we do not communicate with the TV set) where what the child says is attended and responded to. As an example of what *not* to do, we have heard many teachers and speech-language pathologists place such an emphasis on form that the communication intent of the child seemed to be actively discouraged. A child can be asked "where did you go yesterday?" and when he responds "to the park," the teacher or clinician corrects him and says, "No, say I went to the park yesterday." If this correction occurs frequently, the child soon loses interest in the exchange. True, he may imitate the teacher upon her demand, but he does not learn any language rules.

Actually, in the example above, the child's response was quite appropriate. He assumed, correctly, that the teacher and he shared information (who was it that went somewhere and when) and he transmitted in his response the necessary new information (to the park). Unskilled teachers and speech-language pathologists are always asking questions like, "How old are you?", "Where do you live?", "Whose toy is that?" and demanding complete sentences in return, when from a language usage perspective, such demands are incorrect. Knowing when and under what circumstance to employ a grammatical ellipsis (where linguistic items are omitted because both partners in the communication exchange share the information) is an important component of language usage therapy.

speech perception training

In the previous section on audiological management, coverage was limited to factors which provide the child with the maximum potential for detecting the most salient acoustic energy in a speech signal consistent with the limitations imposed by his hearing loss. Auditory management can refer to a program as specific as development of self-monitoring expression of syntactic forms or as general as improving speech reception through the auditory channel. Regardless of the goal, four conditions must be met before the management is begun: appropriate amplification is being used, amplification is functioning properly, auditory cues are available for the child to use based on the aided audiogram, and the child has the potential to make better use of his amplified residual hearing.

At this level of reception, meaning is not directly involved, although we can reasonably expect a child to begin constructing meaningful sound/message associations on his own without explicit efforts on our part. Many children, however, require support in moving from the simple detection level to phonemic perception, particularly for those phonetic elements for which the acoustic saliency is insufficient. Moreover, within a structured therapy format, many need assistance and encouragement in moving from a primarily visual dependency in speech perception to a more auditorily based process. Functioning as they have with reduced auditory input for their entire lives, hard of hearing children often evolve strategies for speech perception which unduly deemphasize auditory dependency. Our intention is not to restrict the speech information available through vision, but to increase their auditory capacity and thereby enhance the total perceptual process.

This goal is not limited to improving the perception of the acoustic product of others' speech, but also to the improved auditory monitoring of their own speech products. Indeed, the processes of speech perception and speech production are reciprocally related, with improvements in one area (whether perception or production) having positive repercussions on the child's status in the other area (Ling 1976; Novelli-Olmstead 1979).

As a matter of fact, in our view all the dimensions of a speech and language management program are interrelated with progress in one facet reciprocally reinforcing or inhibiting progress in another. Much of what we will be discussing in Speech Perception Training is therefore relevant and has already been covered earlier, from a slightly different perspective. The therapeutic process cannot be conducted as a sequential development in which therapy in one speech and language dimension is completed before beginning on another; on the contrary, the therapeutic process is usually characterized as an interweaving of foci in which stress is placed first on one and then another dimension but always bears in mind each child's unique problems and needs.

It is important to note at this point that the principles and procedures we will be describing are primarily applicable only to the school-age hard of hearing child. Analytic exercises and lessons can be focused on this child's observable deficiencies in speech perception in an attempt to improve his auditory functioning. For the preschool child (for whom this book is not designed; see Boothroyd 1982) we view speech perception, or auditory training, as an integral component of the naturalistic approach to speech and language development. For this younger population, we would only cautiously and occasionally employ analytic auditory training "lessons"; such efforts are too often considered as ends in themselves, by both the children and the clinicians, and not interwoven into our primary therapeutic objective with such children—improving their communication skills. For the school-age hard of hearing child, on the other hand, whose continuing development of such skills is being unduly limited by auditory deficiencies, our task is to pinpoint his speech perception problems and attempt to overcome or reduce them.

The existing language base of hard of hearing children enables us to analyze the phonemic errors they make in a simple speech discrimination test. By first improving their ability to discriminate and then identify the acoustic constituents in known language, we are not only enhancing their auditory recognition and speech production facility with these known language items, but we are also setting the stage for continued auditory language growth.

In the general suggestions for speech perception training outlined below, we will begin with the child who needs encouragement and practice to increase his confidence and dependency on the auditory perception of speech by increasing his facility to deal with auditory messages. Our first goal here is to demonstrate to them that they can identify speech signals without the aid of visual clues. Often, this is a revelation to them, particularly as the material gets more difficult, or as new material is introduced.

These new signals are simple words which are part of a closed response set of two or more choices. The next stages require the comprehension of simple to complex verbal utterances, terminating in a focus on those acoustic/phonetic elements which code phonemes the child has difficulty perceiving. At this level of speech perception training, a great deal of cycling back and forth between phoneme perception and language comprehension takes place, since deficiencies in one dimension will set limits to the functioning in the other dimension. The stimuli we use is always speech, either the clinician's, some prepared prerecorded material, or, and frequently very productively, the child's own recorded utterances. A great deal of emphasis is placed on self-monitoring, because we want the child to incorporate the problem phoneme in his own speech, so speech perception and production training are often merged—as they should be. Progress in either of these dimensions can have a salutary effect on performance in the other one, such as when refining a child's production of the /s/ will assist him to recognize the same element in the speech of others.

Invariably, speech perception training also merges with vocabulary and syntax therapy, as for example, when the child realizes that he can use the known linguistic context and the nonlinguistic situation in combination with the auditory perceptions to learn new words and verbal material. As we have already noted, it is therefore not possible to deal with speech perception training for very long without the support and inclusion of speech production and language comprehension.

Beyond the general considerations reviewed in the previous paragraph, the following enumerated steps, or stages, apply. They are not intended to be precisely sequential; even if we could exactly define the stages in auditory development which all children, including hard of hearing ones, should follow, which we cannot, too many variations are introduced by the inter-related difficulties in speech and language displayed by different children to use them successfully. In many of the steps we will be interspersing general principles and specific procedures; our reasoning is that no therapy "recipe" should be divorced from the general principle from which it is derived. Otherwise, therapy becomes sterile and nonproductive in the sense that procedures cannot then be modified to fit a particular situation or child. The steps below, therefore, are offered as a guide, not as a sacrament.

(1) Our first concern in training is to ensure that the child can identify —through his hearing alone—one of several known words in a closed response format. This is not as easy as it may sound; many hard of hearing children object vigorously when the view of the speaker's lips is deliberately obstructed. The two words selected should differ by more than one distinctive feature to make the task easy and to guarantee success.

If the child's performance on the speech discrimination tests indicate that he has difficulty with vowel discriminations, then the words selected should incorporate vowel differences. Usually, however, hard of hearing children have little difficulty with the perception of vowels and, therefore, the first task should require consonantal discriminations of manner and voicing, but not of placement since this is the most difficult discrimination to make. For those children who do have difficulty with vowel perceptions, training should begin with words that differ in the number of syllables and then move to vowel judgments; the essential principle is to begin at a level that the child can master.

The words are printed on flash cards (or pictures or objects can be used with the younger children), and the words are spoken by the clinician while the lips are covered or the child's eyes are lowered. The child is asked to immediately imitate what he hears and then to select the stimulus word. Asking him to imitate strengthens the bonds between perception and production and also provides additional information about the child's speech production difficulties. Since our major objective here is to increase his confidence in his ability to make auditory judgments, a correct imitative production is not necessarily expected at this stage (though it may be later).

(2) When the child successfully and easily makes two-word discriminations, more words are added to the set; the clinician must still select words

that offer choices between consonants that differ in manner, voicing, or blends. To make these word discrimination exercises more interesting to a child—and to keep children on their toes—the clinician can add different response modes, such as asking the child to point to the correct word, write it, put a check by it, circle or underline it. When the child is successfully selecting a word from a set of six or eight, then he should be presented with two, three, or more successive words and required to identify the proper order. Only known words are used at this stage, since as we have already indicated the goal is still as much to convey to him that he can rely on hearing alone for speech perception as it is aimed ultimately toward increasing his auditory abilities.

(3) When the child realizes that speech can be recognized using only his hearing, he can then be exposed to entire utterances of increasing length and complexity on clearly defined topics. For example, several pictures (or objects) can be shown to a child with the clinician describing the one he has to select. The pictures can illustrate action sequences (boy running or walking), various attributes of objects (color, size, location, function), similar actions done by different actors (boy or girl running), different sequences of events and so on. The number of pictures from which the choice is made should gradually be increased as should the complexity of the descriptions.

The child's task is to infer the meaning of the verbal passages; this can be accomplished without his perceiving all the acoustic/phonetic or linguistic constituents. Many children will never be able to discriminate all the elements in a speech signal. What is important to convey to them is their ability to auditorially comprehend a message in spite of missing many of the component parts. Later efforts in speech perception training cycle back to the phonemes they have difficulty perceiving, in an effort to enhance their total auditory capacity. Other variations on this level of listening practice require the child to answer questions on such topics as his family (names, ages, where they live, what they do), interests, and hobbies—on any topic, in other words, for which the child has a great deal of prior information to assist his comprehension of the clinician's utterances.

We do not agree with the auditory training philosophy which holds that training *must* proceed from the smallest, essentially meaningless linguistic elements to larger and larger units that are then supposed to terminate in the child's comprehension of meaningful passages. On the contrary, as in normal language development, the child is concentrating on the meaning of messages delivered to him, and only delves (usually unconsciously and automatically) into the specific acoustic/phonetic and/or linguistic composition when the semantic intention must be clarified. When, as we shall see below, the meaning of a verbal passage depends upon the discrimination of particular elements, such as decoding the difference between "he walks home" and "he walked home," then of course the discrimination between the /s/ and the /t/ must be stressed (but keeping in mind that conversational utterances incorporate other acoustic and alternative cues to deduce the meaning).

The goal of speech perception, however, is primarily a search for meaning and not a step by step construction of elemental and then progressively larger linguistic units toward the final edifice of meaning. When, as above, the child engages in word selection exercises, or below, when the child is exposed to difficult acoustic/phonetic discriminations, the explicit goal remains determination of meaning (on the one hand by increasing the child's awareness of the concept that meaning can be derived from incomplete acoustic signals and on the other hand, by assisting him to resolve linguistic ambiguities with improved acoustic/phonetic perceptions).

(4) The complexity of the listening task can gradually be made more difficult by using such techniques as requiring the child to answer true or false to comments on familiar topics and to respond to simple informational questions. For example, the clinician can ask a child if a "ball is square," "grass is white," "motorcycles have two wheels," or if "basketball games are played with nine players on each side." The length and complexity of the comments and questions are gradually increased, while still keeping in mind the child's interests, maturation level, and language capacities when the specific stimulus items are constructed (example: "Manned space flights reached Mars last year," or "Rock music is played with loud stones").

The type of simple informational questions which should be employed as stimuli require the child to answer such queries as, "What month comes after January?", "What number comes after six, or falls between six and eight?", "Is a polar bear white or green?", or "Which is bigger, an elephant or a mouse?". Such questions are easy to devise and made congruent with a particular child's language abilities. In answering them, the child still does not need to perceive every acoustic/phonetic or linguistic element, although more such information is required for these stimuli than those in the previous stage because they contain less linguistic redundancy (if a key word is missed, the answer will be wrong).

There are any number of variations on this listening task theme; the goal is to gradually increase the length (sentences to paragraphs), acoustic difficulty, and linguistic complexity of the task while keeping the material as relevant and motivating to the child as possible. At first only familiar material should be employed, but when he demonstrates increasing confidence and capacity in his auditory impressions, then unfamiliar words or more difficult auditory tasks can be added (but, at this stage, only in a familiar linguistic or situational context).

The child should begin to realize that he can still learn his lessons when the teacher turns to face the board or somehow covers her mouth. Two such variations enjoyed by children require them to complete a simple crossword puzzle using only auditory clues, or to make a game of following verbal auditory directions. For example:

a) Crossword puzzle:
3-down: A baby cow is called a _____.
6-across: A wolf lives in a _____.

b) Directions: Walk over to the door, turn around two times, hop on one foot, and sit down.

(5) The introduction of a tape recorder or a language master into speech perception training provides the clinician with a very useful therapeutic tool. If possible, the recorded output should be delivered to the child with high quality earphones equipped with an individually modified frequency response, rather than through the internal loudspeaker that the child listens to with his hearing aids. Such an earphone connection prevents frequently poor acoustic conditions existing in the therapy rooms from affecting the quality of the acoustic signal received by the child. It is possible however to use the internal loudspeaker so long as the noise level in the room is monitored. In therapy, while new material or acoustic perceptions are being taught, it is important to provide the child with the highest quality signal possible. Once the linguistic perceptions have been assimilated by the child, he can then use his prior knowledge to predict the presence under adverse conditions of any element which is not acoustically salient. (See Ross 1981, for a detailed discussion of this point).

The initial and easiest tasks require the child to listen to a brief, prerecorded word, phrase, or paragraph while following a written script of the same material. Then, words are deleted from the written version. At first only those words that are easily predictable from the context should be deleted; later, words which are less and less predictable from context, can be eliminated from the written text. The child has to complete the written form by listening to the tape recording. Such a technique can be elaborated with many variations including the assignment of "homework" via cassette tapes. Larger stories of interest and pertinence to the child, such as some of his academic material, can be similarly recorded, leading to the omission from the text of new words that the child has to complete and deduce from the context. Morphological endings that the child has not completely mastered are recorded in context, and the child required to fill in the proper missing ending on the basis of the linguistic context or the auditory perception. Eventually, beginning with short, meaningful sentences, the written script is eliminated and the child is required to answer questions about the content of the recording without any additional cues (for example, who did what to whom?).

This kind of activity forces the child to engage his hearing (and his brain) in the comprehension process. In a reality situation—distinct from the therapy requirements—of course the child will supplement this process with vision, as he should; our goal in therapy, however, is to increase the contribution of the auditory channel in his global comprehension of language. For the hard of hearing child who has already evolved his preferred strategy for speech reception, this may not come naturally. They need help to more fully exploit audition.

This is an example of an incomplete script that corresponds to a tape played for the child. His task is to fill in the blanks based on what he hears.

> For   years, Mr. Smith had   a small   on Oak   . He has
> toys,   , gum,   and   novelties to the   of Oldtown. A
> mall has just   up the   and is   business   from Mr. Smith.
> have   off. He can no   make a   , so he is going to   the
> and sell the   . The   of Oldtown   of his plight and   him
> a

(6) When the child demonstrates that he can comprehend messages just through his hearing, then it is a good stage to begin telephone training. Many severely hard of hearing children are reluctant to use a telephone because they have experienced frequent occasions when it was just too difficult. A telephone is a necessary adjunct to interpersonal communication in our society, and any child who cannot successfully make and take calls is limited in his ability to relate in a normal way with his peers. In a carefully structured therapy situation, the child can converse on the telephone with the clinician (or other children) on preselected topics and thereby ensure a successful experience. Telephone calls immediately after school to the child at home, in which the next appointment or assignment is discussed, convey an aura of reality to telephone communication.

Many hard of hearing children do not know how to properly utilize the telephone attachment on their hearing aids for a magnetic coupling with the telephone; such coupling, when possible, produces a great improvement in reception. Since the hearing aid microphone is bypassed, the gain can be increased to any level without feedback or negative effects of environmental noise. For those telephones that effectively eliminate or reduce the magnetic field around the telephone receiver, portable amplifiers are available which intensify either the acoustic or the magnetic signal (Castle 1979). If a child can comprehend messages through a tape recorder he can also employ a telephone with some important measure of success. For the older hard of hearing child in particular, telephone listening training is intrinsically very motivating. The frequency range limitations of telephones, however, should be kept in mind; ordinarily, they do not transmit frequencies beyond 3000 KHz. The hard of hearing child, therefore, has to be assisted in making the same kind of predictions in these circumstances as normally hearing people do.

(7) In the course of increasing the child's confidence and ability to grasp the meaning of solely auditory utterances, many of the child's problems in specific acoustic/phonetic perceptions will become evident. Such therapeutically derived insights provide a reality supplement to similar information gleaned through formal speech discrimination tests. Even though the emphasis in speech perception training focuses on meaning—the transmission of which is, indeed, the purpose of interpersonal communication—there is a point where this purpose can best be met by increasing the child's ability to make acoustic/phonetic perceptions. For example, if a child has difficulty in recognizing and producing an /s/ phoneme and also does not understand pluralization rules, the training for /s/ should not take place on pluralized words. The child has to proceed from the known to the unknown with only one clearly defined task required of him at any one time (learning how to recognize the /s/ or, if he cannot, teaching him to produce it; then, cycling back to check reception training before teaching him the pluralization rule).

In Chapter Two, Tables 2–1, 2–2, and 2–3 show the kinds of phoneme perception errors which hard of hearing children can be expected to make. Many of them have little difficulty producing a number of these phonemes, such as the /p/ or /b/. Their perceptual confusions are based on the intrinsically weak intensity of many of these phonemes, the fact that they may share many distinctive features, and, particularly (for the child with a high frequency hearing loss), the high frequency spectral composition of most of the problem phonemes.

One place to begin training is to devise discrimination exercises in a closed response set using nonsense syllables as stimuli with the problem phonemes first associated with back vowels (the low second formant will make the task easier for most of the children) in different positions. The task can then be extended to different vowels. This is the one step in which we depart from our insistence in using real words as stimuli, mainly because it is impossible to find a sufficient array of words known by the child to enable him to practice discrimination of some problem phonemes in all vowel environments, diphthong environments, in all positions, and in all consonantal blends. We suggest that the clinician consider requiring the child to repeat the stimuli before he makes the discrimination choice. Indeed, as the child works on this task, it may be pertinent to train him to correct an automatic production of the problem phoneme in all the relevant phonetic environments before proceeding with the next one.

As soon as the child is able to perceive the practice stimuli in nonsense syllables, the focus should shift to similar exercises using familiar words, first in a closed response discrimination task, then in an open set for the identification of the same words. Such discrimination and identification exercises will be very difficult for hard of hearing children and most will never achieve perfect scores. Complete success at this stage should not be a prerequisite to training the child to use linguistic *and* nonlinguistic cues to deduce the meaning of a message. Indeed, by focussing on meaning, by helping the child predict the presence of "something" he cannot auditorially perceive, we may be able to foster his ability to find that "some" thing is there after all.

(8) For those children with the requisite language ability, the clinician may find it desirable to bypass or supplement the suggestions in step 7 above by employing as training stimuli those problem phonemes which also serve as morphological markers. Initially, the task presented to the child should be one of discriminating among contrastive endings, such as /walk, walks/; /walked, walk, walks/; /walk, walks, walked, walking/, and /walk, walks, walked, walking, walker/. Each time a stimuli is presented, the child should be expected to say it correctly before making his choice. Deliberate errors may be introduced (the boy walk slow) with the child required to judge whether the sentence is correct or not and, if not, tell why not.

Depending upon a child's specific problems, the training stimuli can mingle clear-cut phonemic with grammatical marker discriminations. For example, requiring the child to select words from the following set: mat, mass, mast, mask, match, matched, masked, matches, matching, masking, mats, masts, masks, starting with just a few foils and progressively increasing the number of possible choices. Such stimuli should include phonemes which the child has problems perceiving as well as those he can recognize easily to ensure that the task poses a reasonable progression of difficulty for him.

After he can achieve a high level of correct closed-set (that is, multiple choice) discriminations repeating each word as it is spoken, variations can be introduced that require the child to spell the stimulus words or to use them in a sentence. As before, speech production and speech perception training cannot really be separated. Both depend heavily upon the child's capacity to auditorially self-monitor his own utterances, and it is to this topic we shall turn to presently.

Before we do, however, we think it is time to introduce a note of caution into this perhaps implicitly over-optimistic picture of a hard of hearing child's auditory possibilities. Try as we may, we are going to reach limits; the hard of hearing child has a sensory deficiency and no amount of training or auditory management can substitute for physiologically normal hearing. The limits that are reached in a training program should not be a source of contention between the clinician, parents, and the child. If all concerned do their best—consistently and intelligently—any unavoidable residual implications of the hearing loss is a fact of life that must be accepted by all concerned. On the bright side, however, we have absolutely no doubt that the functional limits of the overwhelming majority of hard of hearing children have not been reached. It is, in fact, only in recent years that all the programmatic and auditory ingredients for reaching these limits have been potentially if not actually present. As we move into more and more difficult training exercises, the focus must be on the child's accomplishments and not his failures; functional normalcy (as opposed to normal functioning) is a realistic goal to set for most hard of hearing children.

(9) In a previous step, we have already exposed the child to sentence contrasts and asked him to select the one he hears (example: between "He walks upstairs" and "He walked upstairs" or "He drops the ball" or "He dropped the ball"). These are very difficult discriminations to make without the support of the linguistic and nonlinguistic context, but they are within the potential of many hard of hearing children. Their discriminations can be refined, and their speech production and self-monitoring improved by requiring the child to select from words he himself has recorded. The child is asked to put a variety of such constrasts on tape. The clinician randomly starts the tape at a different point; the child then decides which contrast was played. Such judgments convey to the child the need for precise articulation if perceptual judgments are to be correctly made. He has to listen to himself speak and monitor the correctness of his own utterances. These correct productions help sharpen the child's awareness of what to listen for in his own speech and the speech of others. Because of his hearing loss, he may not be able to detect, for example, many of the acoustic correlates of a morphological ending. But by producing the element correctly, this may focus his attention on alternative acoustic cues such as the reduction in vowel length when a word ends in a voiceless consonant or the changes in vowel transitions accompanying different adjacent consonants or the effects of consonant blends on the duration of a component consonant.

For normally hearing persons these alternative acoustic cues may lack saliency or importance since they can select from a host of other cues. These same acoustic cues can be crucial to the hard of hearing child's perception of speech. One cannot, however, simply verbally define an alternative acoustic cue for a child—such as the effects of the phonetic context on duration —and expect him to consciously capitalize upon it in speech perception. What he needs is a great deal of structured practice in the relevant contrasts (such as between /mat and mask/; /bit and bid/; /mat, mask, and masks/; /write and rice/; /robe, rove, and rode/; and /leaf and lease/). The best such alternative perceptual clue, however, may be the one he himself uses and self-monitors when he produces, in various contexts, a phoneme he has difficulty perceiving.

(10) Another technique that can be used at this stage is to have the child relate a story or an experience into the tape recorder and have him critically listen to it later section by section. In each section (perhaps a few sentences),

the child must evaluate the errors, if any, he has made in speech production. In a spontaneous speech sample, a number of grammatical and articulatory errors will usually occur. The clinician has to resist the temptation to jump in on all of them at the same time. The goal here is to try to get the child to hear his own errors, whatever they are, and self-correct.

The explicit instruction given a child for this exercise would be to listen and judge whether he put the proper endings on words, or used contractions correctly, or completed some other clearly defined goal. The other errors, linguistic and articulatory, are noted by the clinician for a separate focus at another time. (This particular recommendation requires the clinical judgment of the speech and language pathologist; some children are ready for, can tolerate, or prefer a more shotgun approach to making corrections, and in these instances, one should by all means go along with the child.)

(11) The final stage in speech perception training is indistinguishable from our final goals in speech production training; it is for the child to self-correct his own utterances as he speaks. This is accomplished without a tape recorder, simply by engaging the child in conversation. As he makes an error, the clinician says "how's that?" or "what was that again?". The child should clearly understand that the purpose of the conversation is for the evaluation of his ability to monitor his speech productions, and therefore accept the fact that the communication intentions of the utterance is of secondary importance at this time. We want to heighten his concentration, during the therapy session, on the perception and production of his speech. Our goal is to move the child from a conscious concentration on his speech to an automatic self-monitoring process. At this latter stage, the child hopefully knows something is wrong because it sounds wrong, just as a normally hearing child does.

Let us briefly review. We seem to have gone far afield from the conventional concept of "auditory training," as indeed we have. We are dealing with hard of hearing children who are in the process of learning language. All, by our very definition of what constitutes a hard of hearing child, will have an auditory language base of some degree. Many have learned to depend heavily on a consistent, though inadequate, visual system for language comprehension rather than an inconsistent and inadequate auditory impression. Our first task with them is to increase their dependence, confidence, and skill in auditory reception. All people, not just hard of hearing children, focus on the meaning of verbal messages directed to them and do not consciously attend to the various constituents of such messages. This is the primary approach we recommend with hard of hearing children. The quest for meaning, however, is severely affected for many hard of hearing children by limitations on specific acoustic/phonetic perceptions. At this juncture, speech perception training can be conceptualized as an ascending spiral with the analytic emphasis intended to enhance the derivation of meaning, which in turn should improve the child's ability to discriminate and identify phonemes. Speech perception training cannot be really separated from prowess at making linguistic predictions, speech production skills, and an eventual capacity to unconsciously and automatically monitor verbal output. Though treated separately in a training program, with an alternating focus on first one aspect and then another, diverse emphases must be harmonized within a given child.

Several examples of complete programs we have written for specific children that incorporate many of the above steps can be found in Appendix D and E.

speech production training

In the previous section, we made some general comments on speech production training for hard of hearing children, but from a speech perception perspective. In this section, we will be discussing speech production training directly, though, of course, the auditory channel is still expected to play a crucial role in such training. Earlier, we also expressed some reservations regarding the average hard of hearing child's ability to discriminate all the meaningful acoustic distinctions in a speech signal; there are limits to what can be done, though we can certainly set our aspirations higher than is usually the case. In regards to speech production, we can reasonably expect this average hard of hearing child to have intelligible speech, understandable to all native listeners. Some children can demonstrate speech virtually indistinguishable from that of a normally hearing child. For most hard of hearing children, we accomplish our speech production goals through a heavy dependence on audition and self-monitoring. For those for whom we cannot, alternative approaches are available.

The most comprehensive and coherent exposition of all approaches pertaining to the speech development and correction for hearing-impaired children is that described by Ling (1976). No professional working on the speech production of either deaf or hard of hearing children should fail to study and attempt to apply the model and procedures presented in his book. In our work, however, dealing as we do with the hard of hearing and not the deaf child, it is the last stages of his seven stage model that are particularly appropriate, particularly those pertaining to the correction of consonants and—in various blends—within and between words (Ling 1976, pp. 174–175).

The children for whom this book is primarily designed come to the therapy process with an already developed, though deviant, phonological system. For the most part, they can employ suprasegmental patterns, vowels, and dipthongs correctly; their major problems in speech, as reviewed in Chapter Two, relate to consonant and blend articulation. There are, of course, exceptions to this generalization. There are hard of hearing children in regular schools who for one reason or another (initial placement in a segregated setting, severe degree of loss, denial of usable amplification) display speech irregularities in such fundamental dimensions as rhythm, voice, quality, and vowel production in addition to the consonants. For these children, the clinician may have to stress fundamental auditory/vocal monitoring of output (the first stage in Ling's model) before proceeding with the second and third stages (prosody and vowels). Parenthetically, for children who manifest such severe speech production deviances that they cannot be understood by their teachers or peers, one must question whether a fully mainstreamed educational placement is the appropriate one.

The results of the speech evaluation serve as the basis for a program of speech production training planned for each individual hard of hearing child. The average such child will omit consonants, particularly in the final position in words, and omit or distort one component of a blend or an affricate as well as consonants requiring tongue-tip placements. Most children will make more than one error, so a decision has to be made concerning the specific target sound with which to begin training.

Our decisions regarding teaching order are not quite so critical for the elementary school age hard of hearing child as they are for the deaf child with little or no oral speech, but nevertheless some general guidelines are in order. In the review of the literature, we suggested that the speech production errors of hard of hearing children resemble those of younger normally hearing children. This suggests that the natural order of the acquisition of speech sounds should serve generally as the basis for therapeutic intervention. In instances where the child has problems with both the voiced and the voiceless members of a cognate pair, we suggest beginning with the voiced. The clinician should attempt to generalize the correct production of a target sound to other problem sounds which have the articulatory features of manner or place of production in common with the target. In the generalization from an initial to a final stop, however, the clinician should be aware of the large phonetic differences occuring with such a phoneme in the released and unreleased positions. Some fricatives, affricates, and blends are the most difficult and the latest developing sounds in the English language and thus would be among the last targets selected by the clinician. For many, if not most, hard of hearing children, however, these are the sounds with which therapy begins, since they represent the major part of their speech production problems.

Therapy is straightforward. We first determine, in the case of the omission of a final consonant for example, if the child knows and can perceive the presence of the weak, perhaps high frequency, element in a linguistic context, and if not, we begin by focusing on speech perception (again, speech perception and production intertwine). Perhaps, as is often the case, the child can perceive and produce the missing element quite adequately when stimulated, but simply omits it in conversational speech. This child needs a great deal of practice in auditory self-monitoring, using such techniques described earlier as recording the child's utterances and having him listen for the inclusions or omissions of the problem element. Similar procedures should be followed for any child who has the capacity to perceive and produce correctly any consonant or blend he habitually omits or distorts in his everyday speech production.

If a child does not know or cannot produce a correct version of a missing or distorted consonant upon demand, and if an intense regime of speech perception training has only limited success, training should consist in teaching the child the direct production of the problem sound using whatever audition is available plus tactual, kinesthetic, and visual clues (see Chapters 16, 17, and 18 in Ling, 1976, for a detailed description of the relevant procedures). Unlike speech perception training, the initial concentration should be on the correct production in meaningless syllabic contexts. The problem sound should first be taught in the most contrasting vowel contexts (the /i/ and the /oo/). The child must be able to repeat the syllable correctly three or four times per second before proceeding to different positions in the syllable (front, medial, or final, depending upon where therapy began). Then, more adjacent vowels are added, and syllabic drill is made more complex, cutting across different vowels and positions.

When the child is able to effortlessly produce the missing or distorted phoneme or blend in various syllabic contexts, generalizations to meaningful phonological speech may occur spontaneously, or with minimum "reminders" by the clinician. The goal is to assist the child achieve automatic correct production of the target at a phonetic, nonmeaningful level, before introducing the additional cognitive complexity of meaning intended to be conveyed.

After mastery of the phonetic level has been demonstrated, the emphasis in speech production training is placed upon meaningful speech. To assist in the generalization from the phonetic to the phonological level, we may require the child to produce the sound in contrasting, known, real word environments such as /loose/, /lease/, /lice/, and /lace/, or /lose/, /lays/, and /lies/. When this is accomplished, the words are inserted in real sentences—first in a carrier phrase ("the word is /loose/") or ("/loose/ is the word") and then in real sentences in various positions ("There is a /loose/ connection in the hearing aid"). It is important to ensure that when this stage is reached the child knows the meaning of the world and sentence used for speech production training. It is important that the child is not confused about the meaning of the stimuli when our focus is on speech production.

Conversational speech at a normal rate contains a number of phonetic elements which are normally elided or unstressed. While teaching a hard of hearing child to incorporate in his speech sounds which he habitually omits or distorts, we do not want to make him, at the same time, guilty of over-precise articulation (admittedly not a frequent occurrence). This danger can be minimized by attention to the rate of the child's utterances; as he achieves a normal rate of expression, the normal physiological constraints affecting the co-articulation of adjacent phonemes should lead to an acceptable pattern of stress and elisions.

○ CLASSROOM MANAGEMENT

In the chapter on evaluation, we outlined the major points concerning the observation of a hard of hearing child in a regular classroom. Such classroom observations are an important component of a comprehensive performance evaluation. The child spends most of his time in the classroom, and it is there that the major part of his education is, or should be, taking place. The observations we make in a classroom are designed to enhance the total effectiveness of the classroom milieu as it affects the academic, communicative, and social performance of the child. None of them are particularly difficult or esoteric; the value of the structure we provided earlier is that it draws the observer's attention to dimensions they may not otherwise explicitly consider. From the perspective of the speech-language pathologist, the teacher of the hearing impaired, or the educational audiologist, most of what we term "classroom management" is a direct and logical consequence of these observations. In our present discussion, we shall follow the format of the classroom observation outline provided in the chapter on evaluation, and conclude with some considerations related to curriculum and the teaching process itself.

participation of the child in classroom activities and discussions

Consider first the child who *never* raises his hand in response to questions posed to the entire class by the teacher. The likelihood is that he can understand at least some of the questions but feels very insecure about the answers or the intelligibility of his oral resonse. If his language or auditory limitations prevent him from comprehending the majority of the comments and questions in class, and if the provision of an FM auditory training system results in little appreciable improvement, an alternative educational placement should be considered.

Many hard of hearing children are quite aware that their speech is "different." People may turn around and look at them when they talk, and they simply do not want to expose their "difference" in a public fashion. We can recall a high school girl who transferred from a special school into a public high school and who talked only once in class. Thereafter she refused to orally respond to any questions or comments because she felt that she was being ridiculed. Such children can be encouraged to increase their classroom participation by making them a member of a student "team" in a classroom exercise, by first phrasing the questions so that only monosyllabic answers are required, and by calling on them for short oral reading passages to increase their confidence and experience in public oral expressions. If, however, the child does not respond because the material seems to be always beyond him, then an intensive regime of tutoring is called for. On the other hand, the learning and behavioral style of many normally hearing children is such that they naturally adopt a quiescent stance in public. The same may be true of a particular hard of hearing child. This child may know the material and be very well aware of what is going on, but his style is simply to sit quietly and never volunteer. Such a child will, however, usually answer a direct question. The child who does not know the material, or is sensitive about his speech, will attempt to evade responding.

Many hard of hearing children give the impression of knowing more than they do. They are keen observers of their peers (sometimes too keen, as when their eyes are always on their neighbor's papers) and will imitate what the other children do without really understanding the situation. Thus, they may raise their hands when the other children do, laugh when they do, and go along with activities without understanding the directions or the purpose.

Classroom teachers, with twenty-five to thirty children to look after, are frequently not aware that a hard of hearing child is imitating, not comprehending. It is necessary, for example, when the child is always raising his hand when the other children do, to actually call upon the child to answer a question to determine if he is understanding or just imitating. The classroom observer should note the occasions when the child superficially appeared to comprehend and later query the child to determine the level of his understanding. This kind of observation will be an aid in helping the child modify learning strategies he uses.

Classroom discussions are particularly difficult for hard of hearing children. The child may be able to understand the teacher quite well, perhaps by using an FM system and also because he is able to clearly observe the speaker's face, but as soon as rapid exchanges occur between the children, he is lost. He has to hear them with the environmental microphones of an FM auditory trainer or his hearing aids, and thus is subject to interference from the acoustical conditions in the classroom. He is unable to predict the next speaker in exchange and thus he loses valuable visual clues while searching for him. In such instances, he hard of hearing child may simply withdraw from the situation mentally, or perhaps in some cases, attempt to control the discussion in order to predict where it is going.

There are several things we can do to ameliorate this situation. One is to give the child freedom of movement, to permit him to move to a classroom location where he can better observe all the other children. In many typical classrooms, this will be to the right or left front with his chair turned slightly around so that he can observe the entire class. The other possibility is for the teacher to sufficiently control the discussion—by calling on each subsequent speaker by name—to give the hard of hearing child time to observe each speaker's face. Unfortunately, classroom discussions are rarely that controlled. Indeed, many teachers would find such control an imposition on their teaching style. In truth, there is often nothing we can do for a hard of hearing child to enable him to fully cue in and participate in a lively class discussion when a large number of children are involved. Fortunately, this does not happen too often in the younger grades. Beyond this, we have to help the child build sufficient ego strength to accept some unavoidable difficulties and, at the same time, attempt to minimize the psycho-social effect upon him through compensatory activities in areas of proficiency (particular academic subjects, hobbies, sports).

interactions between child and teacher

We can preclude many problem interactions between child and teacher by offering an orientation program on the problems and management of a hard of hearing child prior to the time one is enrolled in class; we can continue to reduce such problems by making "expert" consultation available on a scheduled or on-call basis throughout the school year. We often hear of the few "bad apples" in the teaching profession—the ones who resist having a handicapped child their class and when forced to accept one, do it with visible reluctance. We have met a few ourselves and do not doubt their existence; when we do, we also wonder about their sincerity and effectiveness as a teacher of normal children. *Much* more often, however, the teachers we meet are genuinely interested in educating children; their reluctance to accept a hard of hearing child stems from insecurity. Given the assurance of help, their reluctance disappears, particularly after a successful experience with one such child and assurances of help from knowledgeable professionals.

In observing the teacher-child interactions, we are concerned with the naturalness of their exchange. Does the teacher call upon him as often as upon the other children? A teacher may, unconsciously, fall into a pattern of calling upon him less, because of the extra effort it may take to ensure that the child understands. A teacher may have some difficulty following a hearing-impaired student's speech and may feel that there is not time to request that the child repeat or rephrase an utterance. Moreover, a teacher may not even know how often this pattern of interacting with the child occurs.

Since many hard of hearing children (and children in general) prefer that less demands be made upon them, the relative exclusion of a child in some learning activities may not at all be objectionable to him. He may prefer sitting quietly and day dreaming. It is deceptively easy for such a pattern of interactions between the child and his teachers to develop in the first few months of the school year. Once it has, neither may fully appreciate that a different, and *reduced,* set of expectations is operating. The classroom observer, coming to the situation with a fresh and objective viewpoint, can help the teacher analyze—and thus modify—the verbal interaction patterns that have developed.

Often, when hearing a positive report from a teacher on how a certain hard of hearing child is doing, one can almost hear the unexpressed qualification in their mind, "for a handicapped child." That is, a teacher may be more lenient in grading a child on homework assignments, seat work, or tests, because "it really isn't fair" to expect the hard of hearing child to accomplish as much as a normally hearing one. We have seen instances where a teacher actually gave the answers to seat work or quiz assignments —while trying to help a child work out a problem—and then grade the child's work on the basis of these correct answers. This was not done to deceive anyone, but done in the course of trying to offer a child some intensive classroom assistance. Such teachers will usually not be aware how often such instances occur.

Many teachers will be more lenient when a hard of hearing child displays the "roving eye syndrome" than when one of his classmates do it. We know, and have had reports of, children who have gotten through entire grades on the basis of their neighbor's work. What it comes down to is the standards of academic performance the teacher sets for the hard of hearing child. Set unreasonably low, the dynamics of a self-fulfilling prophecy practically guarantees that the child's subsequent achievements will be lower than it could be.

This is not meant to assert the opposite—that performance standards be set unreasonably high. This latter step is practically a prescription for frustration and a reduced self-image. The child should be expected to perform in accordance with his intellectual potential and somewhere within the range of achievements demonstrated by the majority of his classmates. If this level of achievement cannot reasonably be attained, an alternative program should be investigated.

Practically by definition, a hearing loss is an impediment to oral communication. If it takes patience to deal with a normally hearing child, it will take more patience to deal with a hearing-impaired child. Teachers are human (in spite of occasional reports to the contrary by some children) and some will exhibit visible signs of impatience when trying to communicate a point to a hard of hearing child. Enough such occasions and the child will react by withdrawing, acting out, or just being unhappy and feeling that he is being "picked on." Some of the other children may take the lead from the teacher and also react differently to the hard of hearing child. It is necessary for the teacher to set a positive example when dealing with the hearing-impaired child.

The fact that a child has a hearing loss and wears a hearing aid or an auditory trainer must be openly acknowledged by the teacher, the child, and his classmates. It is there, it cannot be hidden, and must be dealt with simply as a fact of life, as an example of one of the differences characterizing all people. In the beginning of the year, a unit on "health" or "hygiene" can be scheduled, within which sensory or physical disabilities are openly discussed. The child can be encouraged to display his hearing aid to the class and demonstrate how it operates. If the child wears an FM system, a really dramatic demonstration can be made, by having the child go to the far end of the room, or leave it entirely, and carry out a conversation with the teacher or one of the other children. It is appropriate to have all the children in the class listen to the FM unit so as to realize its function.

In an accepting, open atmosphere, references to the child's hearing problem should be made frankly and casually when the situation requires it. We want the child to accept himself as he is, with the hearing loss representing just one constituent personal characteristic in a host of others. If the teachers, and through them, the other children can accept the hard of hearing child in this fashion, it will make his personal acceptance of himself that much easier.

Adaptation of the Teacher's Classroom Style   The observer has to tread very carefully when suggesting that teachers modify their teaching style. Theoretically, all teachers should modify their style to meet the needs of individual children. In practice, however, particularly for experienced teachers, presentation of their material comes close to the heart of their concept of themselves as professionals. In making suggestions regarding teaching style, or in any other area for that matter, the observer cannot come across as one who is dispensing wisdom from some lofty superior perch. In our judgment, the classroom teacher has the most difficult, most important, and most responsible position in the entire educational system. For someone who is not required to minister to the day to day needs of twenty-five or thirty disparate children to come into the classroom and appear to criticize the teacher's best efforts is at best stupid and at worst self-defeating. We cannot emphasize this point strongly enough.

The observer (whether the speech/language pathologist, teacher of the hearing-impaired, or the educational audiologist) has to come across as a collaborator on equal terms with the teachers; both professionals combine their unique insights for the child's benefit. Suggestions offered by the observer should not imply a critical judgment. When offering such suggestions a good place to begin is to ask teachers to describe the child from their perspective, then, with the support of specific observations and the results of the comprehensive performance evaluation, the observer should offer an assessment of the child. It is out of this kind of interchange that positive modifications can occur in the classroom style of the teacher and other less than perfect conditions.

The language used by teachers to present material may be overly complex for some hard of hearing children. Speech may be too rapid or indistinct. Or a teacher may be in the practice of talking to the blackboard or behind a piece of paper. When instructing children in general, it is a good idea to paraphrase verbalizations, simplifying and repeating when the child's language level makes it likely that he will have difficulty. The observer must give the teacher specific examples of the kinds of lingusitic processing problems the child manifests based on the speech/language evaluation, and relate them to the language level of the classroom instruction. We are not suggesting "baby-talk," but a level of oral presentation consistent with the material being offered. We have heard 6th-grade science teachers use language more suited to college sophomores and beyond the actual lesson the child was expected to master.

Periodic verification is necessary to ensure that the child has understood the directions of the material. If all the other children in the class are able to handle the level of language complexity of the teacher's presentation and if the hard of hearing child is unable to comprehend the material, then a lower level class or alternative program should be considered.

New topics should be introduced clearly with a short sentence or a key word so that the child can follow changes in activity. Whenever a new train of thought is beginning, it should be signaled by an explicit comment by the teacher (example: We are now going to talk about Pilgrims). After a new or complex concept has been covered, it should be summarized or repeated. Whenever feasible, visual aids should be used (overhead projectors, captioned filmstrips, movies, pictures). Any new concepts or vocabulary arising from such visual material should be reviewed in advance with the child. Such techniques will not only help the hard of hearing child; they are also appropriate for normally hearing children as well. They provide a clear structure to lessons that the children are receiving.

An exceptionally important visual aid is the use of written instructions and summaries. They should be integrated with the oral presentation of the content material. Together, the oral and written clues will help the hard of hearing child keep on top of his lessons. A simple outline should be placed on the board prior to the lesson or a hand-out outline provided for the hearing-impaired child. Whenever possible, written tests should be administered to make certain that the child understands what is expected of him. The short sentences or key words which introduce new topics should also be written on the board. All homework assignments should also be written on the board and not simply presented orally.

If the child is "daydreaming" or being "obstreperous" during or right after a direction or a lesson is given, the teacher should first try to determine if the child knows what is going on before chastising him. Hard of hearing children need to be disciplined just like their normally hearing classmates, but not for situations over which they have no control. The teacher must encourage hard of hearing children to ask questions to verify or clarify oral presentations. If this occurs often enough, it will offer valuable insights into the difficulties experienced by the child and assist in making the necessary modifications in instructions and approach. With the help of the speech-language pathologist, our goal is to give the teacher a feel for classroom modifications necessary for the child to learn in a regular classroom setting.

It is frequently necessary for the teacher to repeat the answers of other children for the benefit of the hard of hearing child. This does not come naturally to someone who can clearly hear an answer and who would therefore tend to assume that everyone else heard it too. If the answer to some question is simply one or two words, the teacher can acknowledge it by saying, "Yes, that's right, Washington, D.C., is the U. S. capital", or "No, New York City is not the capital." If the answer requires more than several words, or if a comment is needed, the teacher has an opportunity to expand, rephrase, or correct the response for the benefit of the entire class, not just the hard of hearing child. It is possible, in some instances of classroom discussion, for the teacher to summarize several of the comments offered by the normally hearing children and thus keep the hard of hearing child in the picture.

interactions between child and classmates

From the point of view of a child, how he gets along with his classmates and the kind of friendships he develops in and out of school, is more important to him than his relationship with the teacher. His view of himself and his feeling of belonging are much more reflective of his peer relationships than that with the teacher, particularly as he gets older. When working with an older child, we often find that our best efforts are frustrated because the child feels that wearing a hearing aid or an auditory trainer will set him apart and make him "different" from his peers. Objective demonstrations of superior auditory abilities with amplification carry little weight when compared to what the child believes his peers will think of him if he has to employ some device. We can attempt to preclude this kind of misconception in our adolescent hard of hearing children by concerning ourselves with peer relationships when they are younger.

Actually, the best time to observe a hard of hearing child interacting with his classmates is not in the classroom at all, at least not during structured activities. The time to observe him is during recess, lunch, in the hall, or free play. In these unstructured situations, it is possible to estimate his status in the group, how the other children deal with and talk to him. Is he included as a full partner in the games? Does he have a special friend? Do the normally hearing children rarely talk to him, and when they do, is it in whispered or shouted monosyllables, accompanied by many gestures? Normally hearing children unconsciously develop a level and system of communication with a hard of hearing child which, on the basis of their experiences with him, is required to get the message across. Unfortunately, it is the verbal interchanges with his peers that the hard of hearing child is most motivated to understand and respond. If the linguistic sample he receives at these optimal times is impoverished, then he is losing valuable opportunities for crucial language exposures.

It is necessary to know how the child handles these kinds of situations. Does he ask the children to repeat themselves ("what?") or is he content to stay in the dark? Does he have a special "buddy"—one he developed himself or one assigned to him by a teacher—who clues him in to what is going on? Or does he simply withdraw, mentally if not physically, from the situation? Superficially, our concern with how a child gets along with his classmates may appear to have little to do with his education. However, not only do these concerns directly impact upon the child's education, but they may even transcend it. An unhappy, isolated child is not in the most receptive state for learning. He cannot benefit from the natural language environment which surrounds him. He cannot grow to emotional maturity. Under these circumstances, even if the child's academic and communication skills appear adequate, we would consider an alternative educational placement. Every child needs friends. The forced mainstreaming of a child who is socially isolated as a direct consequence of his hearing loss, makes him pay the penalty of our scholarly pretensions (or good intentions).

It is possible for a teacher to help, sometimes circumspectly, sometimes directly. Given the kind of open and relaxed classroom atmosphere we discussed earlier, the teacher can help the normally hearing children modify their linguistic input to the hard of hearing child; they can at least open the door, through small-group activities in the classroom, to more social interactions with the hearing children. Other teachers can be asked to assist through something like a group project in art or physical education in which the hard of hearing child is included. A normally hearing child can be asked to repeat or "translate" directions or games upon request by the hard of hearing child; perhaps, even a few children can be asked to take this "assignment."

There is a fine line to draw, of course, between such an assignment being viewed as a friendly and natural overture by one child to another, or as a definition of an inferior-superior relationship. No child wants to feel that an adult is forcing another child to be his friend. Various kinds of extracurricular activities can be encouraged, optimally those in which only small group interactions are necessary. Most hard of hearing children can function one on one very well, and sometimes with two children. But when the social or communicative group increases to three or more normally hearing children, the conversational exchanges may be too rapid for him to follow. There is just no way in which he is going to be able to keep up with the quips, jokes, and gossip whipping their way around the lunchroom table. Under such circimstances, the child has to either be free to stay or move without any pressure from teachers or clinicians who want to "toughen" him up. It makes more sense to try to plug the child into situations in which he can experience communicative success rather than frustration and failure.

child strategies for learning and processing content material

Although some hard of hearing children can function entirely in the auditory mode, particularly when the teacher is employing an FM system, the majority of them have to capitalize on both visual and auditory clues in order to maximize their reception of speech. This means that they must observe the face of the teacher as she talks. If they are doing this, they cannot also take notes while she is talking. Every time they did, they would miss something the teacher is saying.

The learning situation is more effective for a child if he can concentrate his attention on the teacher and not have to divert it by taking periodic notes. At the same time, notes are an important aid for study and review. The teacher should assign a notetaker who makes copies of his notes available to the hard of hearing child. Carbon paper or special paper, available from a stationery store on which several copies are made with one impression, can be used. This task can be alternated between a number of children who have demonstrated that they take exemplary notes.

We have already recommended that the child be encouraged to ask questions when he does not understand the material. Now it must be determined how he asks these questions. Does he simply say what?", or "I don't understand!", or is he able to formulate specific questions on a specific topic which must be clarified? Children can be helped to ask appropriate questions which pinpoint their problem rather than be left to make some generalized expression of ignorance. Indeed, this is a suitable target for individual therapy by the speech-language pathologist, and is another example of the necessity of a team effort. We must first determine if the child understands enough of the material to even formulate questions.

Many children focus on key words they can comprehend and take large inductive leaps to the presumed meaning of the message. While we want them to use context to deduce meaning, this is not a strategy that can carry them very far when they are exposed to complex syntactic transformations combined with a number of morphological endings. They are also prone to depend upon the nonlinguistic situational cues in decoding utterances—

preferring these kinds of cues rather than putting in the necessary mental effort to comprehend ambiguous or unclear verbal messages. For children who demonstrate such strategies, it may be helpful to interpose a slight delay between the time the message is given them and their required response, to give them a chance to think before they jump to conclusions. They often exhibit the same kind of behavior when doing seat work or when taking a test. They go right to the presumed task with only a cursory glance at the directions.

It is important to note when a child is clearly not paying attention, and to try to determine the underlying reasons. The material may be too difficult; the amplification device may not be working; insufficient preparation may have been given him; the level of the ambient noise may be too high; or, and this is a frequently overlooked possibility, the child may simply be wiped out. Trying to comprehend verbal messages all day with an imperfect linguistic and auditory system is a tiring experience. By early afternoon many hard of hearing children have had it. It would be desirable, if possible, to schedule their linguistically based subjects in the morning and their "specials" in the afternoon. There may be, in other words, an optimal readiness time for learning content material.

The Use of an FM Auditory Training System We have already discussed auditory training systems rather extensively in the auditory management section. Our repetition of this topic at this time is designed to emphasize that an FM system is a classroom, and not a clinical tool, and to permit us to expand on some of the points only briefly mentioned previously.

On entering the classroom, the observer (who can be either the speech pathologist, the audiologist, or the teacher of the hearing-impaired) has to make an estimate of the acoustic conditions as they affect the speech signal received by a child wearing a hearing aid. If the child is normally seated more than six or so feet away from the teacher and if normal classroom activities create a moderately noisy hubbub (say about 60 dB SPL at the child's desk), the acoustic conditions are such that an FM system would be highly desirable.

Now the educational approach has to be analyzed. An FM system will help only if the teacher directs significant verbalizations to the child individually or as a member of a group for some important periods of time. We cannot further define "significant" or "important" in any detail; suffice to say that clinical judgment has to be exercised regarding that nature and length of the material presented under adverse conditions.

Some classrooms, in which a teacher fully conforms to an "open" educational plan, wherein all activities are individually programmed and the child just checks with the teacher as his objectives are met, are not conducive to an effective use of an FM system. In such classrooms, the teacher circulates, talking to each child or small group separately; the teacher may spend only a few minutes with each and then go on to the next one. The amount of switching the FM unit on and off which would have to be done (or perhaps the child for some units) would make for a burdensome chore. Furthermore, an FM device may not even be necessary, since when the teacher does talk to a child, it is possible to move closely to him and thus limit the negative effect of poor classroom acoustics. Most classrooms we have seen, however, practice a combination of small and large group and individual instruction, and thus the possible contribution of an FM system requires a unique judgment in each classroom.

We have not, perhaps, sufficiently emphasized that *each* of the child's classrooms and teachers must be observed. Rarely, even in the early elementary grades, is just one teacher involved with a child. The child may leave his homeroom for "specials", such as art, physical education, music, and shop; he may have different teachers for science, social studies, and language arts. In each one, there may be a different constellation of children, teachers, and interactions. For determining the appropriateness of an FM system, every one of these classrooms and activities must be observed. Recommending a unit for the child's homeroom, and then leaving to chance its use in the other classrooms, is sloppy educational practice. Yet in our experience, it is rare to find a hard of hearing child in a regular school who cannot benefit from and FM auditory training system for at least some important periods during the school day.

There are some relatively easy ways to demonstrate the need and usefullness of and FM auditory training system to a classroom teacher. The first step is to acquire the loan of one for a month's trial period. Ordinarily, this should present little difficulty; manufacturer's represenatives can make this arrangement (if one is not already available in the school system). The unit is fit by the educational audiologist to a child and, while the teacher is observing, live-voice discrimination scores are obtained with both the child's hearing aid and with the FM system, in quiet and in moderate noise, at one foot and ten feet distances from the child. The superiority of the FM system at the ten feet under noisy conditions should be quite clear (and sometimes quite dramatic). As a variation of the above procedure, paragraphs requiring aural comprehension can be read to the child under these same conditions.

During the one month's trial period, the teacher is asked to keep a log in which she notes any changes in the child's behavior while wearing the FM. The child, too, is asked for a report, keeping in mind the difference between cosmetic objections and improved auditory performance. A preliminary step, if the teacher and the administrators are reluctant to try an FM on a child, is to play them prepared audio and videotaped presentations of a child listening through a hearing aid and and FM system under various conditions.

After an FM system is obtained, some one person has to take responsibility for seeing to it that it is properly operating. The homeroom teacher is the logical person to assume this responsibility, since this is the first room the child enters in the morning. This person has to ensure that the child puts it on when appropriate and that it is working correctly. At the same time, it is a good practice to troubleshoot the child's hearing aids, since the child may be switching between the FM system and hearing aids throughout some portion of the school day. The teacher has to ensure that the FM microphone and the receiver unit are plugged into the charger at the end of the school day. This is not a responsibility that the classroom teacher, or any other member of the professional staff, has to assume permanently. Beginning at the third grade, if not sooner for some children, the child himself should be taught to take responsibility for his own auditory trainer and hearing aids. Before this obligation is completely passed on to the child, however, a continued program of verification should be conducted to check that he knows how to do it and that he is doing it right.

It is in this aspect of classroom management that the speech-language pathologist, the educational audiologist, and the teacher of the hearing-impaired, often find their most unambigous welcome. At first, many teachers are reluctant to wear "that thing" around their necks. For most of them, this reluctance is soon dissipated as they see a demonstration of its effectiveness. But even when they do agree to wear the unit, with maybe a little coercion from the principal, reinforced by an IEP statement, they still harbor many doubts regarding their ability to operate it correctly. In our experience, these doubts are well founded, but not because the teacher's are unwilling to learn; it is just that operating an electroacoustical device is not something they have done or feel comfortable doing.

Their acceptance of advice and assistance regarding the proper use and care of the FM unit does not threaten their self-concept as a teacher; the operation of such units played no part in their preservice training curriculum! Helping a teacher use an FM system correctly can open doors for effective cooperation in classroom management areas that do bear directly on the teaching process as they see it. Throughout this book, we have stressed the overriding need for the proper auditory management of hard of hearing children. Determining the necessity for an FM auditory trainer, and ensuring that teacher's use it correctly, will go a long way in helping make this goal a reality.

The following outline is a summary of the important observations to make regarding how an FM auditory training system is used in an school setting:

1. Does the teacher turn the FM microphone off when presenting material not intended for the hard of hearing child to hear or when what is being said is not pertinent to the child at that time?

2. Does the teacher pass the microphone to another child who is called upon —for example, the child speaking during show and tell. When this is not possible, does the teacher repeat the salient information?

3. Is the FM system being used when a talk is given by someone who is not the teacher—for example, in the auditorium?

4. Often an FM system is not possible to use during physical education; does the teacher ensure that the child has heard the instructions?

5. In some noisy classroom situations—for example, shop—it may be advisable to turn off the environmental microphone and only direct information to the hard of hearing child via the teacher microphone.

6. With audio-visual equipment, the best way to use the FM system is via the auxiliary input jack. In doing so, it is necessary to ensure that the external speaker of the equipment is not overridden. If the equipment is designed so that the external speaker is shut off when the auxilary jack is used, then the teacher should place the FM microphone close to the loudspeaker (but taking into considering the equipment noise).

7. The teacher and the child should devise an unobstrusive signal whereby the child can indicate when the teacher microphone is not activated—for example, child points to microphone.

8. The teacher should visually check the child's unit several times during the school day to ensure that the settings are correct—for example, reception from the teacher microphone. This helps make the child ultimately responsible for the operation of the unit.

Source, Level, and Location of Speech and Noise Sources   Not all children who need them are fortunate enough to have the use of an FM auditory training system to minimize the negative effect of classroom acoustics; even for those that do possess one there are many times during the school day when its use is not educationally appropriate. We must therefore go about identifying and measuring the noise sources in a classroom, the child's proximity to a noise source, the estimated relationship between the speech and the noise at the child's location, and what steps we can take to reduce noise and increase the speech to noise ratio.

By keeping eyes and ears open, a classroom observer can easily identify the sources of noises in the classroom. Many of these are internally developed in the classroom; some sounds are transmitted into the classroom by external sources. Many of them are such a routine component of the educational milieu that normally hearing people hardly pay attention to them unless they show periodic variations or their intensity increases markedly.

Hearing-impaired children, however, will find such "commonplace" noises a significant impediment to the comprehension of speech. The constant drone of an air conditioner or a steam hiss escaping from a radiator; the motor of a movie, slide, or overhead projector; the constant scraping of chairs and tables; the not-so-muted hum of children engaged in learning activities all are normal intrinsic noise accompaniments to the classroom process and tend to be ignored or accepted. Ths sounds produced on hard

floor corridors right outside the room, those created in adjacent gymnasi-
ums, lunch rooms, or other activity rooms, windows open on a busy street
or playground are all extrinsic sources of noise transmitted into the classroom. While their presence may be noted, they are often accepted with a
fatalistic resignation, for it is felt that nothing can be done about them.

The first step in reducing the level or the source of the noise is to first
convince the teacher and the school administrators of their deleterious
effect upon the hard of hearing child. The data presented in Table 4–6 offer
an objective demonstration of the effects different levels of noise and reverberation have upon word discrimination scores for both normally hearing
and hard of hearing children with and without hearing aids. In itself, however, we have found that such a demonstration does not always make a
convincing argument; it seems too remote from the child in question. Making measurements with a sound-level meter, such as shown in Table 4–5
helps, but also does not seem to be sufficient.

What we have found most convincing is to record speech through a
child's hearing aid right in the classroom and then play it back to the teacher.
A simple device for doing this was described by Randolph (1976). Basically,
a rubber crutch or chair tip is placed over the microphone of a cassette
recorder to form an approximate 2 cc cavity. A plastic L–shaped tubing is
inserted in the tip; ear-level aids are inserted right into the tubing while a
plastic adapter can be used for body aids or FM receiver units. During
normal classroom activities, the aid is removed from the child's ear and
inserted into the make-shift coupler. All sounds entering the microphone of
the hearing aid are recorded on the tape recorder. When played back, the
recording permits the teacher to gain some insight into how noise and
speech is processed through a hearing aid. The subjective effect is that of
a great increase in noise relative to the speech, with more of an increase the
further the speech source is from the microphone. Prepared tapes of this
kind of auditory experience can be played to teachers during their orientation sessions, and periodically reinforced by on-site recordings. Such a
demonstration, coupled with the objective data referred to above, is usually
sufficient to sensitize the classroom teacher to the unwelcome effects of
noise upon the reception of speech by a hard of hearing child.

When identified, the hard of hearing child should be seated as far away
from the noise source as possible—consistent of course with also hearing
the teacher and the other children in an optimum fashion. The IEP can
specify modifications in the room so as to make the acoustic environment
more suitable for a hard of hearing child. We know of instances where a rug
was obtained for a classroom because of the needs of one hard of hearing
child.

We do not yet know of examples where such major provisions as acoustic
tile, silent air conditioners (to keep from opening a window on a busy
street), or sound baffles in heating and air conditioning ducts were included

in an IEP and made available for a hard of hearing child (see discussion on the IEP). Based on our reading of Public Law 94–142, however, in which "architectual" modification must be made for a handicapped child, we do not see any logical reason why such a provision should not be extended to the needs of a hard of hearing child as well. As we indicated earlier, however, in the section on "auditory managment," there are also a number of simple and inexpensive steps which can be taken to make the classroom acoustical environment more suitable for such a child.

The point of all of this is to ensure that the child receives the teacher's speech in a highly favorable relationship to the noise, that is the speech to noise ratio should exceed 15 to 20 dB. We are not suggesting that the teacher shout above the level of any existing noise level, after we have done what we could to reduce it. In most classroom situations, the teacher can move close to the hard of hearing child while giving instructions or lessons to the class. If the child cannot clearly hear the teacher at a suitable level above the background noise, he is not very likely to learn the material, (at least from the classroom presentation).

Academic Considerations We expect a hard of hearing child in a regular classroom to follow the curriculum prescribed for that class. As long as he is mainstreamed with normally hearing children, our expectancies are that his academic performance must justify this placement. We do not expect him necessarily to demonstrate average achievements in all his subjects, but he should fit in existing groups within the classroom (Northcott 1979). Major changes in the curriculum should not be necessary and are not appropriate.

The necessity for such changes would bring into question the suitability of the child's placement. Within each regular hearing classroom we expect to see a range of academic achievements, spanning three to four years with the children often grouped for different activities depending upon their ability. The hard of hearing child should be able to perform adequately within this grouping arrangement. We make this point because regular teachers and administrators sometimes request a special curriculum for a hard of hearing child, or express their reservations about enrolling such a child in a regular class because they assume that major curriculum modifications must be made. Such misconceptions seem to be based on their categorizing hard of hearing children with deaf children in special classes, who do follow a revised curriculum (though if a "deaf" child is also fully mainstreamed, he too should follow the regular curriculum).

We do expect, however, that the hard of hearing child will require extra assistance to enable him to follow the prescribed curriculum. Many normally hearing children also require a tutorial program to bolster their academic performance. Their need for such extra assistance does not jeopardize their enrollment in a regular class nor should it for a hard of hearing child. The most effective tutoring program for this child includes a preview, teach, and review paradigm. According to Birch (1976), every successful mainstream program for hearing-impaired children he surveyed included this arrangement. In this procedure, the academic tutor reviews prospective lessons with the classroom teacher who then gives the child a preview of coming attractions by discussing the content, emphasizing new concepts and language with simplified examples. After the classroom teacher presents the lessons (the "teach" component), the tutor reviews the material to ensure that it has been mastered by the child.

The speech-language pathologist has a major role to play in this endeavor. Many, if not most, of the child's problems at the preview stage are going to involve new vocabulary or more complex linguistic structures. Speech-language pathologists are the professionals whose training has specifically prepared them in these areas of a child's deficiencies. For those children whose overall academic performance is satisfactory, an enriched program of language therapy may be all the extra tutorial assistance they require. In case of any doubt, though, we should not hesitate to strengthen the child's supportive program by employing the services of an academic tutor or a teacher of the hearing-impaired.

For those children who are performing satisfactorily, there may be a suggestion by some school administrators that the tutoring service be withdrawn from the hard of hearing child. The budget pie can only stretch so far and there are undoubtedly other needy children in the school system. This would be, in our judgment, an inadvisable step to take. The fact that a hard of hearing child is doing well is a demonstration of the efficacy of the total supportive program; withdraw one component of it, and his performance is likely to get worse. A hard of hearing child is not in the same position as a normally hearing child with special needs who, once his performance is adequate, can function with the rest of his class without extra assistance. The needs of the hard of hearing child will, for most such children, persist right through to high school at least. Since their hearing is not going to get any better, they are going to continue to miss much auditory/verbal material, and, therefore, the compensatory program must continue.

It is sometimes a good policy to have the first or second grade hard of hearing repeat a grade, even if his overall academic performance superficially appears to be adequate. The objective support for such a judgment is based on the child's language/communication abilities. In these early grades, academic demands are frequently concrete and analytical, and the hard of hearing child may appear to do quite well. If the child, however, demonstrates serious deficiencies in the language assessment, then the impact will begin to be felt at the third, fourth, and higher grades. The child may need the extra year in the lower grade to prepare him for the linguistic demands to come.

The social/emotional factors also have to be considered. If such a child is completely integrated with the same peer group, in and out of school, the repetition of a grade could be a painful blow to his self-esteem; we would prefer in such instances, to try a really enriched therapeutic program before taking such a step. On the other hand, for the hard of hearing child who has only a marginal acceptance with his peer group, the repetition of a grade can bolster his self-esteem. He would be a little older than his classmates, perhaps with capacities (nonlinguistic) that they do not yet possess, and his previous experiences may help him find a desired niche among his new classmates. The fact that he already knows much of the work should make a positive adjustment to the new class that much easier. We just raise the possibility of this step here; the taking of it is, of course, a highly individualized judgment.

○ THE EDUCATIONAL AUDIOLOGIST

A pervading theme in this book has been the necessity for providing hard of hearing children with knowledgeable and continuing auditory management in the schools. By now a reader may legitimately protest "enough already, the point has been made!" We must, however, beg the reader's indulgence just a little longer, even at the risk of overkill. The entire rationale we have presented, all of our good intentions, will come to nought if the school system lacks the trained personnel to oversee the sophisticated implementation of auditory management.

Speech-language pathologists possess, actually or potentially, many of the required competencies. Just about all school systems in the United States employ these professionals. They have a direct and crucial role to play as regards total management of hard of hearing children in the regular schools. Nevertheless, when they are available, and we want to make the case now that they should be employed in every school system (sometimes on a regional basis), educational audiologists are the ones whose specialized competencies make them the most suitable professional to oversee a school based comprehensive audiological management program. In the last few years we have noted that an increasing number of these individuals are being employed by public school systems. This is a heartening development and one that has to be nurtured and encouraged—most effectively by the actual demonstration of their necessity to the local and state school officials.

The alternative to having an on-site educational audiologist is to continue to depend upon the availability of audiological services from a physically and administratively separate center, with a great deal of effort expended trying to work out a mutually acceptable working relationship. Although motivated and competent professionals can employ such a model with a fair degree of success, there are inherent contradictions to this arrangement which no amount of good will or skill can completely overcome.

The child has to be taken from school and transported to an audiology center. There he has to be "registered"; many forms have to be filled out, and ongoing records must be kept in several offices; arrangements must be made through one or more agencies for the payment of the services, often with the time-consuming help of professional social workers; a communication exchange (written, phone, or personal visits) must be initiated between the center and the school. This latter necessity is more often a disaster than not (as we have elucidated in the section on audiological management). These redundant, and often unnecessary administrative requirements, add a financial burden to society, with no consequent benefits and indeed a loss of efficiency to the child receiving the services. This occurs because we have engaged an administratively separate agency to provide what are basically educational services.

There are other disadvantages in depending upon outside centers in providing audiology services to hearing-impaired children. The child may not be able to bring his auditory training system to the clinic because either he—or someone—forgot to bring it home the night before for a morning appointment in a physically separate clinic or because school officials are reluctant to let school property be taken home. Often, too, clinic-based audiologists may not even know that the child uses such a unit. Visits by these audiologists to the schools are difficult to arrange; the school must compensate the clinic for the visit, but are reluctant to pay for the travel time involved. The clinics, on the other hand, are not in a position to continually absorb the cost of the time it takes for the audiologist to travel to the school and back (which usually involves cancelling one or more other appointments). Rarely, therefore, are such visits scheduled on a continuing and frequent basis.

The day to day audiological emergencies which never cease occurring, such as the onset of sudden feedback with an aid or auditory trainer, an inoperable hearing aid or auditory trainer, or a change in the auditory responsiveness of the child take an inordinate amount of time to deal with when a knowledgeable person is not immediately available. The speech-language pathologist or, when one is employed by the system, the teacher of the hearing-impaired, should be able to solve many of these day-to-day emergencies, but not the more involved ones (such as the need to make a temporary earmold, administer impedance audiometry, troubleshoot an FM system or its recharger, or run an electroacoustic analysis of the hearing aid). For these kinds of problems, audiological expertise is required at the site they occur.

We should recall that clinic-based audiological management of children was not a planned event; it was not deliberately created as a model to care for the audiological needs of hearing-impaired children. Such a model evolved as an outgrowth of the development of audiology centers focussing mainly on adults. The children were simply plugged into the existing possibilities, while all concerned tried to do the best job they could under prevailing constraints. Now, however, we must acknowledge the technological developments of a new era and marshall them for the benefit of hearing-impaired children. In our judgment, this is impossible to accomplish without trained on-site personnel to oversee their utilization. We must, in other words, organize a new programmatic model—one which brings current technological developments right into the schools. The educational implications of proper audiological management cannot be realized in absentia.

Audiological management of all hearing-impaired children begins when we detect them. While for the "deaf" child, the effects of the loss cannot easily be overlooked until they start school, the hard of hearing child's first confirmation of hearing loss often occurs after he begins school. So the educational audiologist is the logical person to supervise the school system's program for identification audiometry (see Wilson and Walton 1978, for a comprehensive description of such a program). This function should not be underestimated, particularly now that we have more insight into the potential effects of even mild and intermittent hearing losses (Katz 1978; Kessler and Randolph 1979).

A properly organized hearing conservation program—incorporating as it does the training of personnel, the calibration of equipment, the keeping of appropriate records, and the provision of an efficient follow-up program— is a time consuming and involved process. The contribution that educational audiologists can make to the school system by supervising such a program can be used as an entree point to justify to school officials the need to employ one. The economics of the situation can help lend additional weight to this argument.

Each child who fails the screening examinations must receive a more comprehensive audiometric evaluation. The cost for a large number of these evaluations are borne by the school, certainly for those children at least whose IEP states that audiometric tests be administered to them. In this category, one will find children with a history of chronic otitis media, and those found to be developmentally disabled or exhibiting other "special" needs. The IEP of every child who wears a hearing aid, as well as those who do not, but manifest a significant loss should include the necessity for at least a yearly comprehensive audiological evaluation. All this costs money. Though we doubt that an educational audiologist will ever recoup his cost by administering such tests within the framework of a school system, nevertheless the continuing expense of creating an educational audiology position may not be as high as it would seem to be at first. Ultimately, of course, the most urgent justification must be educational; if we cannot defend such a position on educational grounds, no other reasoning would be accepted.

The greatest initial expense in employing an educational audiologist is the need to provide him with the tools he must have in order to do the job. The extent to which he can carry out his detailed responsibilities—as covered in the sections on audiological assessment and management—depends upon the equipment and facilities available. The less the audiologist has available in the school system, the more contracting with outside centers will be necessary. This arrangement is a bit unwieldy, but it can be moderately effective since the on-site audiologist is in a good position to collaborate on equal professional terms with a clinic-based audiologist.

In these instances, the school audiologist acts as the initiator, controller, traffic manager, and interpreter regarding any outside audiological assistance required. The more complete facilities are available to the educational audiologist, the less outside contracting will be necessary. A complete public school audiological center should be indistinguishable from the average outside audiology clinic. It should include a sound-treated two-room testing suite, a two-channel clinical audiometer, one or more portable audiometers, an impedance bridge, an electroacoustic hearing aid analyzer, an octave-band sound-level meter (incorporating an audiometer calibration unit preferably), a stock of loaner hearing aids and FM auditory training systems, a complete set for taking ear impressions, including insta-mold capability, battery testers, and hearing aid stethescopes. Most of these are capital expenses; once purchased, they should last for years (provided a budget is included for periodic repair). It is not necessary to duplicate the medical audiology capacity of some outside centers and include provisions for electro-physiological auditory tests.

The actual delivery of the audiological services can be expedited, at a great savings in time, efficiency, and convenience for all concerned, if the audiological equipment and facilities were incorporated in a mobile audiometric van. This would permit the services to be brought to the children, rather than the other way around. Such a van would not only be useful in rural areas, but in urban locations as well, if children who require attention are not found in one immediate geographic area (such as would be true in the case of an "educational park"). The school system's hearing conservation program could also be greatly simplified if a mobile audiometric van were employed.

Our judgment is that any school system which enrolls 8000 or more pupils requires and can justify the need for a full-time educational audiologist. Providing audiological services to this number of children is a full-time job. Actually we think it is more than a full-time job, but it takes time to accept a new idea. Once on the job, the educational audiologist is in a position to demonstrate a significant contribution to the educational process and thereby support recommendations for the intensification of the services provided. Let us consider the extent of these responsibilities with a school population of this size.

Each year about 2000 of the children will receive a hearing screening. The personnel who actually perform the screening have to be supervised, the equipment has to be functioning properly, records of failure and referral have to be kept. Of the 2000, perhaps 5 to 10% will fail the screening tests, of which 3 to 5% require individual testing by the audiologist, or about 60 to 100 such tests a year.

The demographic data reviewed in the first chapter indicate that 15 to 30 per 1000 school children will have a hearing loss in excess of 16 dB in their better ear. Taking the minimum figure, we can estimate that about 120 children (15% of 8000) will show this degree of loss and require some individual tests each year. This population would only overlap in part with those identified through hearing screening; thus we can estimate about 200 complete evaluations each year. Many of the younger children with known, and significant losses, must be monitored more than once a year.

Of the population of 8000 children, we can also assume that about 100 will have or require amplification. Many will be using a binaural fitting. The educational audiologist must therefore administer between 100 and 200 behavioral and electroacoustic hearing aid evaluations each year. All the children who wear amplification should be considered potential candidates for an FM auditory training system. We realize that this will appear to be a revolutionary, or at least unreal, recommendation for many persons; we make it on the basis of the hard of hearing child's auditory needs, and not the existing "reality" (our goal in managing such children is to improve this "reality" and not sanctify it). Therefore, the classroom conditions and the educational approach for each of these children must be evaluated for a possible FM system recommendation. Speech-language pathologists, classroom teachers, and children must be trained to troubleshoot their amplification systems. Additionally, the educational audiologist who serves as the IEP case coordinator has taken on what is turning out to be an extraordinarily time-consuming task—not just the clerical work involved—but all of the necessary and continuing contacts that must be made with school personnel and parents.

What we have outlined above is clearly a full-time job. Moreover, it is not a clinical job, as this term is generally understood, but one which places the communicative and educationals needs of hard of hearing children foremost. Educational audiologists cooperate with their medical colleagues. When a child fails a school screening, when the hearing loss appears to be progressive, when an impedance battery suggests a middle ear problem, they must not only recommend an otological examination, but keep abreast of the situation to ensure that the recommendation has been followed. Nevertheless, their primary purpose cannot be defined in medical terms; their specialty is the nonmedical habilitation of hearing-impaired children. Among their responsibilties is the sensitization of their medical colleagues to the communicative, educational, and psycho-social implications of a hearing loss. The resolution of a child's middle ear problem, for example, cannot proceed casually, with appointments every several weeks or months to check on progress. The child will miss too much in the interim.

The educational audiologist is a new creature on the educational scene. They will be met with suspicion and confusion ("don't audiologists work in hospitals and test hearing?"); their contribution to the educational process will not be immediately appreciated. Those who work in schools now are literally pioneers; it is doubtful if more than a handful had another educational audiologist precede them in their current position.

In short, this new specialty has to sell itself and its professional contributions. Whatever most of the personnel in the school know about educational audiology will be through the efforts of the educational audiologist. If this person fouls up, it is not just a personal failure, but one which will bring the whole concept of educational audiology into disrepute. And more importantly, the audiological management of hard of hearing children would remain wedded to an antiquated and ineffective model.

This book is intended to provide information to assist speech-language pathologists, teachers of the hearing-impaired, and educational audiologists to work with hard of hearing children in regular schools. These children are seen to manifest deficiencies in speech, language, and academic performance that are clearly related to their hearing losses; furthermore, the evidence indicates that, within broad limits, the severity of their deficiencies is related to the severity of their hearing losses. The need for a comprehensive performance evaluation, prior to planning or implementing therapeutic intervention, was strongly stressed. A recurring theme in the book was that this therapeutic intervention must begin with the provision of appropriate audiological management—taking into consideration such factors as speech acoustics, classroom acoustics, electroacoustics, FM auditory training systems, and the child's hearing loss. Once these factors are optimized for a child, then the therapeutic implications of the rest of the performance evaluation can be considered.

Professionals working with hard of hearing children should keep in mind that of all types of children who manifest communication disturbances, these children probably show the most promising prognosis for improvement. Unlike many other children with speech, language, and educational problems, the cause of their difficulties is known, and remediation measures are clear-cut. In the past, the hard of hearing child has been forgotten (except by himself and his family, of course) and caught between two worlds, the deaf and the hearing. The point of view we have taken is that these children are more like hearing children than they are like deaf children, and that, allowing for minor modifications, the curriculum and expectations they are exposed to should be similar to those their normally hearing peers are exposed to. Given appropriate management in all respects, hard of hearing children are capable of a normal range of achievements and a normal range of contributions to the society when they grow up; our hope is that professionals can manifest the same capacity for growth inherent in the children and that they will employ this book for that purpose.

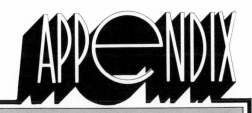

APPENDIX

○ A KINDERGARTEN PB WORDS

○ B EXAMPLES OF LETTERS JUSTIFY-
ING THE NEED FOR AN FM AUDITORY
TRAINING SYSTEM

○ C SENTENCES FOR THE PERCENT IN-
TELLIGIBILITY PROCEDURE

○ D EXAMPLES FOR IMPROVING SELF-
MONITORING SKILLS

○ E EXAMPLE OF SPEECH PERCEPTION
TRAINING FOR THE PHONEME CON-
TRASTS /EE/ AND /OO/, AND /T/ and
/K/

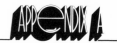

○ KINDERGARTEN PB WORDS

List 1

1. please	14. rag	26. smile	39. dish
2. great	15. put	27. bath	40. neck
3. sled	16. fed	28. slip	41. beef
4. pants	17. fold	29. ride	42. few
5. rat	18. hunt	30. end	43. use
6. bad	19. no	31. pink	44. did
7. pinch	20. box	32. thank	45. hit
8. such	21. are	33. take	46. pond
9. bus	22. teach	34. cart	47. hot
10. need	23. slice	35. scab	48. own
11. ways	24. is	36. lay	49. bead
12. five	25. tree	37. class	50. shop
13. mouth		38. me	

List 2

1. laugh	14. turn	26. path	39. got
2. falls	15. grab	27. feed	40. as
3. paste	16. rose	28. next	41. grew
4. plow	17. lip	29. wreck	42. knee
5. page	18. bee	30. waste	43. fresh
6. weed	19. bet	31. crab	44. tray
7. gray	20. his	32. peg	45. cat
8. park	21. sing	33. freeze	46. on
9. wait	22. all	34. race	47. camp
10. fat	23. bless	35. bud	48. find
11. ax	24. suit	36. darn	49. yes
12. cage	25. splash	37. fair	50. loud
13. knife		38. sack	

List 3

1. tire	14. else	26. most	39. white
2. seed	15. nest	27. thick	40. frog
3. purse	16. jay	28. if	41. bush
4. quick	17. raw	29. them	42. clown
5. room	18. true	30. sheep	43. cab
6. bug	19. had	31. air	44. hurt
7. that	20. cost	32. set	45. pass
8. sell	21. vase	33. dad	46. grade
9. low	22. press	34. ship	47. blind
10. rich	23. fit	35. case	48. drop
11. those	24. bounce	36. you	49. leave
12. ache	25. wide	37. may	50. nuts
13. black		38. choose	

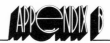

○ EXAMPLES OF LETTERS JUSTIFYING THE NEED FOR AN FM AUDITORY TRAINING SYSTEM

May 7, 1979

J   C
Speech Clinician
Windham Center School
Windham, CT   06280

Re: L   D

Dear Ms. C   :

Your student, L   D   , appears to be a good candidate
for a wireless FM amplification system. This system, used
only in school, enables a child to receive direct auditory
stimulation from the teacher while suppressing environmental
noise.

In light of L   's hearing loss and his dependence on proper
amplification for receiving a strong auditory signal, an
FM system would be most appropriate.

Although the hearing aids he is wearing provide the proper
amplification in most situations, the school setting is a
very special one. In this setting, L   needs to be able
to attend to what the teacher and/or the other students are
saying without being distracted by environmental noise. The
wireless FM system allows for such a condition as well as a
"hearing aid" condition when appropriate.

It is my recommendation that an FM wireless system be purchased so that L   can begin to use it. You have a list
of available dealer's addresses which we gave you in
September. If you have any questions please call me or D   .

Sincerely,

A   M   , Ph.D.
Project Co-Director
UConn Mainstream Project

AM:sg

October 31, 1978

Ms. L   I   , M.A.
Speech-Language Clinician
Fuller School
619 Main Street
Somers, CT   06071

                                      Re: W   D

Dear L   ,

    Your student, W   D   , appears to be in a class-
room situation which would benefit from physical modifications
to improve the classroom acoustics. Such modifications include carpeting on the floor, drapes on the windows and
acoustic tiles on the walls and ceilings. It should be noted
that while the average environmental noise level in a classroom is typically 60 dB SPL, the noise level measures which
were made in W   's classroom on October 3, 1978 demonstrated noise levels of 60-75 dB SPL. Such levels make it
difficult for him to receive good auditory signals.

    An alternative from these physical changes in the room
would be the use of an FM wireless auditory trainer. This
system, used only in school, enables a child to receive
direct auditory stimulation from the teacher while suppressing environmental noise. In light of W   's hearing loss
and his dependence on proper amplification for receiving a
strong auditory signal, an FM system would be appropriate.

    Although the hearing aids he is wearing provide the
proper amplification in most situations, the noise levels
in the school setting make it difficult for him to hear even
with his hearing aids. Through the physical changes made to
his classroom and/or an FM auditory trainer W   would be
better able to attend to the teacher and other students
without being so distracted by environmental noise.

    I hope this information is of benefit to you in meet-
ing W   's unique educational needs. If there are any
questions please feel free to contact me.

Sincerely,

A   M   , Ph.D., CCC-A
Project Co-Director
UConn Mainstream Project

AM:sg

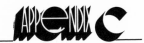

○ SENTENCES FOR THE PERCENT INTELLIGIBILITY PROCEDURE

1. "Bread"
   "Thread" is the first word.
   "Red"
   "Bed"

2. Bring me my ball
                bowl
                bell
                bow.

3. She will write "mouse"
                   "clown" for you.
                   "crown"
                   "mouth"

4. Which one is the neck
                     desk
                     nest
                     dress?

5. Write the word "knee"
                   "tea" now.
                   "key"
                   "bee"

6. The pan
        fan is over there.
        can
        man

   We can see the school
                   broom
                   moon
                   spoon·

8. He saw the fox
               socks there.
               box
               blocks

9. Write "eye"
          "pie" in the book.
          "fly"
          "tie"

10. The |chick / stick / dish / fish| is on the floor.

11. Is the |shirt / church / dirt / skirt| over there?

12. He said the word |"wing" / "string" / "spring" / "ring"| next.

13. Let her see the |floor / door / corn / horn.|

14. She took the |straw / dog / saw / frog| from me.

15. |"Stair" / "Bear" / "Chair" / "Pear"| is easy to say.

16. Show me the |gun / thumb / sun / gum.|

17. I can spell the word |"arm" / "barn" / "car" / "star."|

18. He saw the |train / cake / snake / plane| there.

19. Help me look for the |bus / rug / cup / bug.|

20. The |smoke / coat / coke / goat| is outside.

21. What does |"hat" / "flag" / "bag" / "black"| start with?

22.

He wants to see the $\begin{vmatrix} \text{pail} \\ \text{nail} \\ \text{jail} \\ \text{tail.} \end{vmatrix}$

23.

Did she say $\begin{vmatrix} \text{"wheel"} \\ \text{"seal"} \\ \text{"queen"} \\ \text{"green"?} \end{vmatrix}$

24.

Color the $\begin{vmatrix} \text{ship} \\ \text{lip} \\ \text{crib} \\ \text{bib} \end{vmatrix}$ red.

25. $\begin{vmatrix} \text{"Street"} \\ \text{"Meat"} \\ \text{"Feet"} \\ \text{"Teeth"} \end{vmatrix}$ is the last word.

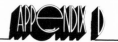

○ EXAMPLES FOR IMPROVING SELF-MONITORING SKILLS

1) Child selects which word is said to him:
walked   walk
walked   walks
walked   walk   walks   walking
Contrast *with other endings,* with someone else saying them.

2) Put in a sentence that could accommodate at least two of the forms, so that you have a contrast:
he walked upstairs
he walks upstairs
Have the child select the one that he hears.

3) Have the child select the same options presented on audio tape or language master. Make sure that the machine can reproduce good high frequencies.

4) Have child tell if the sentence you put on the tape is correct. If wrong, why? Child has to listen for endings in order to do this task:
He walk up the stairs yesterday

5) Child puts a variety of contrasts on a tape. You start the tape at random and see if child knows which one *he* has said.

6) Have child talk into the recorder for a few minutes and then evaluate his own endings, correct or not.

7) Next step is monitoring own speech while he is saying it with help from outside person saying "How's that?"

8) Last step is self-correction because it sounds wrong when it is said.

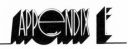

○ EXAMPLE OF SPEECH PERCEPTION TRAINING FOR THE PHONEME
CONTRASTS /EE/ AND /OO/, AND /T/ AND /K/

1. Analysis of errors.
2. Contrast errors:
   a) ee   oo
   b) T   K
3. Contrast in different consonants and vowels:
   bee   boo
   eeb   oob
   eet   oot
   Put into words:
   beet
   boot
   bait
   bite
   Then into sentences:
   I see the_____.
   _____.
   _____.

4. Many contrasts in one sentence:
   John watched the beet
        washed   boot
        walked   bait

5. Use endings to contrast:

wash	walk	cat	cats
washed	walked	book	books
washes	walking	bone	bones
washing	walks	wall	walls
		cup	cups

6. Sentences to contrast endings:
   He washed the car.
   He washes the car.

7. Started to use tape recorder for homework, in:
   ____crossword puzzles
   ____word-finding puzzles
   ____questions about pictures
   ____math problems

8. Cloze procedure (more closely resembles the inconsistent signal the teacher gets in school).

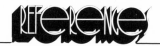

American National Standard Specifications for Audiometers. 1969. S3.6. American National Standards Institute [ANSI], New York.

ARTHUR, G. 1952. *The Arthur Adaptation of the Leiter International Performance Scale.* Psychological Service Center Press, Washington.

BAKER, H. and LELAND, B. 1959. *Detroit Tests of Learning Aptitude.* Bobbs-Merrill Co., Indianapolis.

BINNIE, C. A., MONTGOMERY, A. A. and JACKSON, P. L. 1974. "Auditory and Visual Contributions to the Perception of Consonants," *J. Speech Hear. Res.* 17, 619–630.

BIRCH, J. W. 1976. *Hearing-Impaired Children in the Mainstream.* Publication of the Leadership Training Institute/Special Education, University of Minnesota. Council for Exceptional Children, Reston, Va.

BLOOM, L. and LAHEY, M. 1978. *Language Development and Language Disorders.* John Wiley & Sons, New York.

BOOTHROYD, A. 1976. *The Role of Hearing in Education of the Deaf.* Clarke School for the Deaf, Northampton, Mass.

BOOTHROYD, A. 1978. *"Speech Perception and Sensorineural Hearing Loss,"* in *Auditory Management of Hearing-Impaired Children,* Ross, M. and Giolas, T. G., eds., University Park Press, Baltimore.

BOOTHROYD, A. 1982. *Hearing Impairments in Young Children.* Prentice-Hall.

BOYLE, PATRICIA. 1977. *Psychology in Hearing Loss in Children.* B. Jaffe, ed., University Park Press, Baltimore, 266–282.

BRANNON, J. and MURRY, T. 1966. "The Spoken Syntax of Normal Hard of Hearing and Deaf Children," *J. Speech Hear. Res.* 9, 604–610.

BRANNON, J. B. 1968. "Linguistic Word Classes in the Spoken Language of Normal, Hard of Hearing and Deaf Children," *J. Speech Hear. Res.* 11, 279–287.

BYERS, V. B. 1973. "Initial Consonant Intelligibility by Hearing-impaired Children," *J. Speech Hear. Res.* 16, 48–55.

CARROW, E. 1973. *Test for Auditory Comprehension of Language.* Learning Concepts, Austin, Texas.

CARROW, E. 1974. "A Test Using Elicited Imitation in Assessing Grammatical Structure in Children," *J. Speech Hear. Disord.* 39, 437–444.

CASTLE, D. 1979. "A Growing Need: Resources for Information about Signaling Devices for the Hearing-impaired," *Hearing Instruments,* 80, July.

CLOPTON, B. M. and WINFIELD, J. A. 1976. "Effect of Early Exposure to Patterned Sound on Unit Activity in Rat Inferior Colliculus," *J. Neurophysiol.* 39, 1081–1089.

CLOPTON, B. M. and SILVERMAN, M. S. 1977. "Plasticity of Binaural Interaction. II. Critical Period and Changes in Midline Response," *J. Neurophysiol.* 40, 1275–1280.

COSTA, C., MALAT, R. and MAXON, A. B. 1980. "A Comparison of Soundfield Aided Thresholds to Coupler-predicted Thresholds in Children," paper presented at the American Speech-Hearing-Language Association Annual Convention, November 1980, Detroit.

COX, R. M. 1979. "Acoustic Aspects of Hearing Aid–Ear Canal Coupling Systems," in *Monographs in Contemporary Audiology*, Schwarts, D. M. and Bess, F. H., eds., 1, No. 3.

DALSGAARD, S. C. and JENSEN, O. D. 1976. "Measurement of the Insertion Gain of Hearing Aids," *J. Audiol. Tech.* 15, 170–183.

DALZELL, J. and OWRID, H. L. 1976. "Children with Conductive Deafness: A Follow-up Study," *Brit. J. Audio.* 10, 87–90.

DAVIS, J. 1974. "Performance of Young Hearing-Impaired Children on a Test of Basic Concepts," *J. Speech Hear. Res.* 17, 342–351.

DAVIS, J. and BLASDELL, R. 1975. "Perceptual Strategies Employed by Normal-hearing and Hearing-impaired Children in the Comprehension of Sentences Containing Relative Clauses," *J. Speech Hear. Res.* 18, 281–295.

DICARLO, L. M. 1968. "Speech, Language, and Cognitive Abilities of the Hard-of-hearing," in *Proceedings of the Institute on Aural Rehabilitation*, SRA Grant, #212–T–68, University of Denver, 45–66.

DUBLINSKE, S. and HEALEY, W. 1978. "PL 94–142: Questions and Answers for the Speech-Language Pathologist and Audiologist," *Asha* 20, 188–205.

DUBLINSKE, S. 1978. "PL 94–142: Developing the Individualized Education Program (IEP)," *Asha* 20, 380–397.

DUFFY, J. K. 1967. "Audio-visual Speech Audiometry and a New Audio-visual Speech Perception Index." Maico Audiological Series, Volume V, Report 9.

DUGAL, R. L., BRAIDA, L. D., and DURLACH, N. I. 1980. "Implications of Previous Research for the Selection of Frequency-Gain Characteristics," Chapter 17, in *Acoustical Factors Affecting Hearing Aid Performance*, Studebaker and Hochberg (Eds.), University Park Press, Baltimore.

DUNN, L. 1965. *Peabody Picture Vocabulary Test (PPVT)*. American Guidance Service, Circle Pines, Minn.

DURRELL, D. and HAYES, M. 1969. *Durrell Listening-Reading Series (Intermediate Level): Combined Listening and Reading Tests.* Harcourt, Brace, Jovanovich, New York.

ELLIOT, L. L. 1967. "Some Possible Effects of the Delay of Early Treatment of Deafness," *J. Speech Hear. Disord.* 10, 209–224.

ELSER, R. P. 1959. "The Social Position of Hearing Handicapped Children in the Regular Grades," *Except. Child.* 25, 305–309.

ERBER, N. P. 1974. "Visual Perception of Speech by Deaf Children: Recent Developments and Continuing Trends," *J. Speech Hear. Disord.* 39, 178–185.

FINITZO-HIEBER, T. and TILLMAN, T. W. 1978. "Room Acoustics Effects on Monosyllabic Word Discrimination Ability for Normal and Hearing-impaired Children," *J. Speech Hear. Res.* 21, 440–458.

FISHER, A. and LOGEMAN, J. 1971. *Fisher-Logeman Test of Articulation Competence.* Houghton-Mifflin, Geneva, Ill.

FLAVELL, JOHN. 1975. *The Development of Role-Taking and Communication Skills in Children.* Robert E. Krieger Publishing Co., Huntington, N.Y.

FRY, D. B. 1978. "The Role and Primacy of the Auditory Channel in Speech and Language Development," in *Auditory Management of Hearing-Impaired Children,* Ross, M. and Giolas, T. G., eds., University Park Press, Baltimore.

GAETH, J. H. 1967. "Learning with Visual and Audiovisual Presentations, in *Deafness in Childhood,* McConnell, F. and Ward, P. H., eds., Vanderbilt University Press, Nashville.

GEMMILL, J. E. and JOHN, J. E. J. 1975. " A Study of Samples of Spontaneous Spoken Language from Hearing-impaired Children," *Teach. Deaf.* 75, 193–201.

GENGEL, R. 1971. "Acceptable Speech to Noise Ratios for Aided Speech Discrimination by the Hearing Impaired," *J. Aud. Res.* 11, 219–222.

GENGEL, R. W. 1974. "Mean Intelligibility Functions of Nine Sensorineural Hearing-impaired Ss for vowels and Consonants," in Stark, R. E., ed., *Sensory Capabilities of Hearing-Impaired Children,* University Park Press, Baltimore, 131.

GERBER, S. 1974. *Introductory Hearing Science.* W. B. Saunders Co., Philadelphia.

GOLD, T. and LEVITT, H. 1975. *Comparison of Articulatory Errors in Hard of Hearing and Deaf Children.* Communication Sciences Laboratory, Graduate School and University Center, City University of New York.

GOLDMAN, R., and FRISTOE, M. 1969. American Guidance Service, Circle Pines, Minn.

GOODGLASS. H., BERKO, J., BERNHOLTZ, N. and HYDE, M. 1972. "Some Linguistic Structures in the Speech of a Broca's Aphasic," *Cortex* 8, 191–212.

GOTTLIEB, M. E., ZINKUS, P. W., and THOMPSON, A., 1979. "Chronic Middle Ear Disease and Auditory Perceptual Deficity," *Clinical Pediatrics,* 18, 725–732.

HAMP, N. W. 1972. "Reading Attainment and Some Associated Factors in Deaf and Partially Hearing Children," *Teach. Deaf.* 70, 203–215.

HAMILTON, P. and OWRID, H. L. 1974. "Comparisons of Hearing Impairment and Socio-cultural Disadvantage in relation to Verbal Retardation, *Brit. J. Audio.* 8, 27–32.

HARFORD, E. R., 1980. "Techniques and Applications in Hearing Aids; The Use of a Miniature Microphone in the Ear Canal for the Verification of Hearing Aid Performance," *Ear and Hearing,* 1, 329–337.

HAWKINS, D. B. 1980. "Loudness Discomfort Levels; A Clinical Procedure for Hearing Aid Evaluations," *J. Speech. Hear. Disord.* 45, 3–15.

HINE, W. D. 1970. "The Attainments of Children with Partial Hearing," *Teach. Deaf* 68, 129–135.

Hiskey-Nebraska Test of Learning Aptitude. Union College Press, Lincoln, Nebraska.

HOLM, V. A. and KUNZE, L. H. 1969. "Effect of Chronic Otitis Media on Language and Speech Development," *Pediatrics* 43, 833–839.

JENSEMA, C. J. 1975. *The Relationship between Academic Achievement and the Demographic Characteristics of Hearing Impaired Children and Youth.* Office of Demographic Studies, Gallaudet College, Series R, No. 2.

JENSEMA, C. J., KARCHMER, M. A. and TRYBUS, B. J. 1978. *The Rated Speech Intelligibility of Hearing Impaired Children: Basic Relationships and a Detailed Analysis.* Office of Demographic Studies, Gallaudet College, Series R, No. 6.

JENSEMA, C. J. and TRYBUS, R. J. 1978. *Communication Patterns and Educational Achievement of Hearing Impaired Students.* Office of Demographic Studies, Gallaudet College, Series T, No. 2.

KATZ, J. 1978. "The Effects of Conductive Hearing Loss on Auditory Function," *Asha* 20, 879–886.

KENNEDY, P., NORTHCOTT, W., McCAULEY R. and WILLIAMS, S. N. 1976. "Longitudinal Sociometric and Cross-sectional data on Mainstreaming Hearing Impaired Children: Implications and Preschool Programming," *Volta Rev.* 78, 71–82.

KESSLER, M. and RANDOLPH, K. 1979. "The Effects of Early Middle Ear Disease on the Auditory Abilities of Third Grade Children," *JARA* 12, 6–20.

KILLION, M. C. 1980. "Problems in the Application of Broadband Hearing Aid Microphones," in *Acoustical Factors Affecting Hearing Aid Performance*, Studebaker and Hochberg, (eds.), University Park Press, Baltimore.

KLEFFNER, F. R. 1973. "Hearing Losses, Hearing Aids, and Children with Language Disorders," *J. Speech Hear. Disord.* 38, 232–239.

KODMAN, F., JR. 1963. "Educational Status of Hard-of-hearing Children in the Classroom," *J. Speech Hear. Disord.* 28, 297–299.

LECKIE, D. 1979. "Pilot Study of the Effects of Early Auditory Training on Speech Perception by Profoundly Deaf Children," paper presented at Voice Conference, Toronto, May 26, 1979.

LEE, L. 1974. *Developmental Sentence Analysis.* Northwestern University Press, Evanston, Ill.

LENNEBERG, E. H. 1967. *Biological Foundations of Language.* John Wiley & Sons, New York.

LEONARD, L. B., PRUTTING, C. A., PEROZZI, J. A. and BERKLEY, R. M. 1978. "Nonstandardized Approaches to the Assessment of Language Behaviors," *Asha* 20, 371–379.

LEVITT, H. 1978. "The Acoustics of Speech Production," in *Auditory Management of Hearing-Impaired Children.* Ross, M. and Giolas, T. G., eds., University Park Press, Baltimore.

LEVITT, H. and RESNICK, S. B. 1978. "Speech Reception by the Hearing-impaired: Methods of Testing and the Development of New Tests," *Scand. Audio.* Suppl. 6, 107–130.

LIBERMAN, A. M., COOPER, F. S., SHANKWEILER, D. P. and STUDERT-KENNEDY, M. 1967. "Perception of the Speech Code," *Psychological Review* 7, 431–461.

LING, D. 1978. *"Personal Communication."* Comment in discussion summary in *Auditory Management of Hearing-Impaired Children,* M. Ross and T. G. Giolas eds., University Park Press, Baltimore.

LING, D. and LING, A. H. 1977. *Basic Vocabulary and Language Thesaurus for Hearing-Impaired Children.* A. G. Bell Association, Washington.

LING, D. 1978. "Auditory Coding and Recoding: An Analysis of Auditory Training Procedures for Hearing-impaired Children," in *Auditory Management of Hearing-Impaired Children,* Ross, M. and Giolas, T. G., eds., University Park Press, Baltimore.

LING, D. 1976. *Speech and the Hearing-Impaired Child: Theory and Practice.* A. G. Bell Association, Washington.

LING, D. 1978. *Teacher/Clinician's Planbook and Guide to the Development of Speech Skills.* A. G. Bell Association, Washington.

LUTERMAN, D. 1979. *Counseling Parents of Hearing-impaired Children.* Little, Brown and Company, Boston.

MARKIDES, A. and ARYEE, D. T. K. 1978. "The Effect of Hearing Aid Use on the User's Residual Hearing," *Scand. Audio.* 7, 19–25.

MARKIDES, A. 1978. "Whole-word Scoring versus Phoneme Scoring in Speech Audiometry," *Brit. J. Audio.* 12, 40–50.

MARKIDES, A. and D. T. K. ARYEE, 1980. "The Effect of Hearing Aid Use on the User's Residual Hearing. II. A Follow-up Study," *Scand. Audiol.* 9, 55–80.

MARTIN, F. 1978. *Pediatric Audiology,* Prentice-Hall, Englewood Cliffs, N.J.

MASTERS, L. and MARSH, G. E., 1978. "Middle Ear Pathology as a Factor in Learning Disabilities," J. Learning Dis. 11, 54–57.

McCLURE, A. T. 1977. "Academic Achievement of Mainstreamed Hearing-impaired Children with Congenital Rubella Syndrome," *Volta Rev.* 79, 379–384.

McNAMARA, K. 1980. "An Alternate Procedure for Syntax Assessment of Hearing impaired Children," presented at American Speech-Hearing-Language Association Convention, Detroit, November 1980.

McDONALD, E. 1968. *McDonald Deep Test of Articulation.* Stanwix House, Pittsburgh.

MONTGOMERY, G. W. G. 1967. "Analysis of Pure-tone Audiometric Responses in Relation to Speech Development in the Profoundly Deaf," *J. Acoust. Soc. Amer.* 41, 53–59.

MONSEN, R. B. 1978. "Toward Measuring How Well Hearing-impaired Children Speak," *J. Speech Hear. Res.* 21, 197–219.

MORGAN, D., DIRKS, D. and BOWER, D. 1979. "Suggested Threshold Sound Pressure Levels for Frequency Modulated Tones in the Sound Field," *J. Speech Hear. Disord.* 44, 37–54.

NEEDLEMAN, H. 1977. "Effects of Hearing Loss from Early Recurrent Otitis Media on Speech and Language Development," in *Hearing Loss in Children: A Comprehensive Text.* Jaffe, B., ed., University Park Press, Baltimore, 640–649.

NORTHCOTT, W. H. 1979. "Implications of Mainstreaming for the Education of Hearing-impaired Children in the 1980's," paper presented at the National Technical Institute for the Deaf, 10-year anniversary colloquia, Rochester, N.Y.

NORTHERN, J. L. and DOWNS, M. P. 1978. *Hearing in Children,* 2nd edition. Williams and Wilkins, Baltimore.

OLLER, D. K. and KELLY, C. A. 1974. Phonological Substitution Processes of a Hard of Hearing Child," *J. Speech Hear. Disord.* 39, 64–74.

OLMSTEAD-NOVELLI, T. 1979. "Production and Reception of Speech by Hearing-impaired Children," unpublished M.S. thesis, School of Communication Disorders, McGill University, Montreal.

OLSEN, W. O. 1977. "Acoustics and Amplification in Classrooms for the Hearing Impaired," in *Childhood and Deafness: Causation, Assessment and Management.* Bess, F., ed., Grune and Stratton, New York.

OWENS, E. 1978. "Consonant Errors and Remediation in Sensorineural Hearing Loss," *J. Speech Hear. Disord.* 43, 331–347.

PASCOE, D. P. 1975. "Frequency Responses of Hearing Aids and their Effects on the Speech Perception of Hearing-impaired subjects," *Ann. Otol. Rhinol. Laryng.* 84, Suppl. 23.

PASCOE, D. P. 1978. "An Approach to Hearing Aid Selection," *Hear. Instrum.* 29, 12–16, 36.

PATCHETT, T. A. 1977. "Auditory Pattern Discrimination in Albino Rats as a Function of Auditory Restriction at Different Ages," *Dev. Psychol.* 13, 168–169.

PAUL, R. L. and YOUNG, B. 1974. *The hard of hearing child in the regular classroom.* ESEA Title Project, Oakland Schools, Pontiac, Michigan.

PAUL, R. L. and YOUNG, B. 1975. "The Child with a Mild Sensorineural Hearing Loss; The Failure Syndrome," paper delivered at the International Congress on Education of the Deaf, Tokyo.

PECKHAM, C. S., SHERIDAN, M. and BUTLER, N. R. 1972. "School Attainment of Seven-year Old Children with Hearing Difficulties," *Develop. Med. Child Neurol.* 14, 592–608.

POLLACK, D. 1970. *Educational Audiology for the Limited Hearing Infant.* Charles C Thomas, Springfield, Ill.

PRESSNELL, L. 1973. "Hearing-impaired Children's Comprehension and Production of Syntax in Oral Language," *J. Speech Hear. Res.* 16, 12–21.

PREVES, D. A. and GRIFFING, T. S. 1976. "In-the-ear Aids: Part I, II, III and IV," *Hearing Instruments* 77, No. 3, 5, 7 and 9.

Public Health Service Publication. 1964. No. 1227, 43–44.

QUIGLEY, S. P. and THOMURE, R. E. 1968. *Some Effects of Hearing Impairment upon School Performance.* Institute for Research on Exceptional Children, University of Illinois.

QUIGLEY, S. P., SMITH, N. L. and WILBUR, R. B. 1974. "Comprehension of Relativized Services by Deaf Students," *J. Speech Hear. Res.* 17, 325–341.

QUIGLEY, S. P., WILBUR, R. B., POWER, D. S., MONTANELLI, D. S. and STEINKAMP, M. W. 1976. *Syntactic Structures in the Language of Deaf Children.* Institute for Child Behavior and Development, Urbana Ill.

QUIGLEY, S. P. 1978. "Effects of Hearing Impairment on Normal Language Development," in *Pediatric Audiology,* Martin, F., ed., Prentice-Hall, Englewood Cliffs, N.J., 35–63.

RANDOLPH, K. 1976. "Checking Hearing Aid Operation Using a Cassette Recorder," *Audio. and Hear. Ed.* 2, 28–29.

ROGERS, W. T., LESLIE, P. T., CLARKE, B. R., BOOTH, J. A. and HORVATH, A. 1978. "Academic Achievements of Hearing Impaired Students: Comparisons among Selected Populations," *B. C. Journal of Special Education* 2, No. 3, 183–209.

REICH, C., HAMBLETON, D. and HOULDIN, B. K. 1977. "The Integration of Hearing Impaired Children in Regular Classrooms," *Amer. Ann. Deaf* 122, 534–543.

ROSENBERG, P. E. 1966. "Misdiagnosis of Children with Auditory Problems," *J Speech Hear. Disord.* 31, 279–283.

ROSS, M. 1964. "The Variable Intensity Pulse Count Method (VIPCM) for the Detection and Measurement of the Pure-tone Thresholds of Children with Functional Hearing Losses," *J. Speech Hear. Disord.* 29, 477–482.

ROSS, M. and MATKIN, N. 1967. "The Rising Audiometric Configuration," *J. Speech Hear. Disord.* 32, 377–382.

ROSS, M. and CALVERT, D. R. 1967. "The Semantics of Deafness," *Volta Rev.* 69, 644–649.

ROSS, M. and LERMAN, J. W. 1970. "A Picture Identification Test for Hearing Impaired Children," *J. Speech Hear. Res.* 13, 44–53.

ROSS, M. and GIOLAS, T. G. 1971. "Effect of Three Classroom Listening Conditions on Speech Intelligibility," *Amer. Ann. Deaf* 116, 580–584.

ROSS, M., KESSLER, M. E., PHILLIPS, M. E. and LERMAN, J. W. 1972. "Visual, Auditory, and Combined Mode Presentations of the WIPI Test to Hearing Impaired Children," *Volta Rev.* 74, 90–96.

ROSS, M., DUFFY, R. J., COOKER, H. S. and SERGEANT, R. J. 1973. "Contribution of the Lower Audible Frequencies to the Recognition of Emotions," *Amer. Ann. Deaf* 118, 37–42.

ROSS, M. 1976. "Assessment of the Hearing Impaired Prior to Mainstreaming," in *Mainstream Education of Hearing Impaired Children and Youth*, Nix, G., ed., Grune and Stratton, New York.

ROSS, M. 1977. "A Review of Studies on the Incidence of Hearing Aid Malfunctions," in *The Condition of Hearing Aids Worn by Children in a Public School Program*, HEW Publication No. (OE) 77–05002.

ROSS, M. 1978. "Classroom Amplification," in *Hearing Aid Assessment and Use in Audiologic Habilitation*, Hodgson, W. R. and Skinner, P. H., eds., Williams and Wilkins, Baltimore.

ROSS, M. and GIOLAS, T. G. 1978. "Introduction," chapter 1 in *Auditory Management of Hearing-Impaired Children: Principles and Prerequisites for Intervention*, University Park Press, Baltimore, 1–13.

ROSS, M. 1978. "Mainstreaming: Some Social Considerations," *Volta Rev.* 80, 21–30.

ROSS, M. 1978. "Classroom Acoustics and Speech Intelligibility," in *Handbook of Clinical Audiology*, 2nd edition. Katz, J., ed., Williams and Wilkins, Baltimore.

ROSS, M. and GIOLAS, T. G. 1978. "Issues and Exposition," in *Auditory Management of Hearing-Impaired Children*, eds., University Park Press, Baltimore.

ROSS, M. 1980. "Binaural vs. Monaural Amplification," in *Binaural Hearing Aids*, Libby, ed., Zenetron, Inc., Chicago.

ROSS, M. 1981. "Personal versus Group Amplification; The Consistency vs. Inconsistency Debate," in *Amplification for Education*, Bess, F., ed., A. G. Bell Association, Washington.

SANDERS, D. 1965. "Noise Conditions in Normal School Classrooms," *Except. Child* 31, 344–353.

SEEWALD, R. and ROSS, M. 1978. "Communication Modes of Hearing-impaired Children," paper presented at 1978 ASHA convention, San Francisco.

SEEWALD, R. C. 1981. "The Interrelationships among Hearing Loss, Utilization of Auditory and Visual Cues in Speech Reception and Speech Production Intelligibility in Children," Ph.D. dissertation, University of Connecticut.

SHEPARD, D. C., DeLAVERGNE, R. W., FRUEH, F. X. and CLOBRIDGE, C. 1977. "Visual-neural Correlate of Speechreading Ability in Normal-hearing Adults," *J. Speech Hear. Res.* 20, 752–765.

SILVERMAN, M. S. and CLOPTON, B. M. 1977. "Plasticity of Binaural Interaction. I. Effect of Early Auditory Deprivation," *J. Neurophysiol.* 40, 1266–1274.

SKINNER, M. W. 1976. "Speech Intelligibility in Noise-induced Hearing Loss: Effects of High-frequency Compensation," unpublished Ph.D. thesis, Washington University, St. Louis.

Standard for Specification of Hearing Aid Characteristics. 1976. S322. American National Standards Institute, New York.

STEER, M. D., HANLEY, T. D., SPUEHLER, H. E., BARNES, N. S., BURK, K. W. and WILLIAMS, W. G. 1961. *The Behavioral and Academic Implications of Hearing Losses among Elementary School Children.* Purdue Research Foundation, Project No. P.U. 2040.

STARK, R. E., ed., 1974. *Sensory Capabilities of Hearing-Impaired Children.* University Park Press, Baltimore.

STUDEBAKER, G. A. and WARK, D. J., 1980. "Factors Affecting the Intelligibility of Hearing Aid Processed Speech." Paper presented at the annual meeting of the American Speech-Language-Hearing Association, Detroit.

SUBTELNY, J. 1975. "An Overview of the Communication Skills of NTID Students with Implications for Planning of Rehabilitation," *J. Acad. Rehabil. Audiol.* 8, 33–50.

SUMBY, W. H. and POLLACK, I. 1954. "Visual Contributions to Speech Intelligibility in Noise," *J. Acoust. Soc. Amer.* 26, 212–215.

TEES, R. C. 1967. "Effects of Early Auditory Restriction in the Rat on Adult Pattern Discrimination," *J. Comp. Physiol. Psychol.* 63, 389–393.

TEMPLIN, M. and DARLEY, F. 1969. *Templin-Darley Tests of Articulation,* 2nd edition. Bureau of Education Research and Services, University of Iowa.

THORUM, ARDEN. 1980. *Fullerton Language Test for Adolescents.* Consulting Psychologists Press, Palo Alto, California.

TILLMAN, T., CARHART, R. and OLSEN, W. 1970. "Hearing Aid Efficiency in a Competing Speech Situation," *J. Speech Hear. Res.* 13, 789–811.

TRYBUS, R. J. and KARCHMER, M. A. 1977. "School Achievement Status of Hearing Impaired Children: National Data on Achievement Status and Growth Patterns," *Amer. Ann. Deaf* 122, 62–69.

VILLCHUR, E. 1978. "Signal Processing," in *Auditory Management of Hearing-Impaired Children.* Ross, M. and Giolas, T. G. eds., University Park Press, Baltimore.

WEBSTER, D. B. and WEBSTER, M. 1977. "Neonatal Sound Deprivation Affects Brain Stem Auditory Nuclei," *Arch. Otolaryngol.* 103, 392–396.

Wechsler Intelligence Scale for Children (WISC). 1974. Phychological Corporation, New York.

WEST, J. J. and WEBER, J. L. 1973. "Phonological Analysis of the Spontaneous Language of a Four-year-old, Hard-of-hearing Child," *J. Speech Hear. Disord.* 38, 25–35.

WHITEHEAD, R. L. and JONES, K. O. 1976. "The Influence of Consonant Environment on Duration of Vowels in the Speech of Normal Hearing, Moderately Hearing Impaired and Deaf Adults," paper delivered to the 92nd meeting of the American Acoustical Society.

WILCOX, J. and TOBIN, H. 1974. "Linguistic Performance of Hard of Hearing and Normal Hearing Children," *J. Speech Hear. Res.* 17, 286–293.

WILSON, W. R. and WALTON, W. K. 1978. "Public School Audiometry," in *Pediatric Audiology,* Martin, F. N., ed., Prentice-Hall, Englewood Cliffs, N.J.

WILSON, G. W., ROSS, M. and CALVART, D. R. 1974. "Experimental Study of the Semantics of Deafness," *Volta Rev.* 76, 408–414.

YOUNG, D. and McCONNEL, F. 1957. "Retardation of Vocabulary Development in Hard of Hearing Children," *Except. Child* 23, 368–370.

ZINKUS, P. W., GOTTLIEB, M. I. and SCHAPIRO, M. 1978. "Developmental and Psychoeducational Sequelae of Chronic Otitis Media," *Amer. J. Dis. Child* 132, 1100–1104.

ZINKUS, P. W. and GOTTLIEB, M. I. 1980. "Patterns of perceptual and academic deficits related to early chronic otitis media," *Pediatrics.* 66, 246–253.